Preparing for the Athletic Trainers' Certification Examination

Second Edition

Lorin Cartwright, MS, EMT, ATC
Pioneer High School, Ann Arbor, Michigan

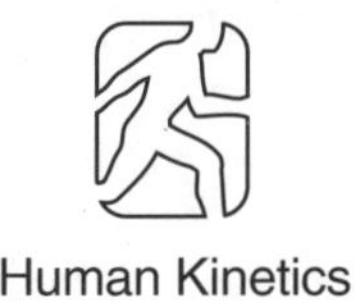

Library of Congress Cataloging-in-Publication Data

Cartwright, Lorin, 1956-
Preparing for the athletic trainers' certification examination / Lorin Cartwright.--2nd ed.
p. cm.
Includes bibliographical references.
ISBN 0-7360-3453-6
1. Personal trainers--Certification--Examinations--Study guides. I. Title.

GV428.7 .C37 2002
613.7--dc21

2002017319

ISBN: 0-7360-3453-6

Acquisitions Editor: Loarn Robertson; **Developmental Editor:** Jeff King; **Assistant Editors:** John Wentworth and Kim Thoren; **Proofreader:** Jim Burns; **Graphic Designer:** Nancy Rasmus; **Graphic Artist:** Kathleen Boudreau-Fuoss; **Cover Designer:** Keith Blomberg; **Printer:** Versa Press

Printed in the United States of America 10 9 8 7 6 5 4 3 2 1

Human Kinetics
Web site: www.humankinetics.com

Europe: Human Kinetics, Units C2/C3 Wira Business Park, West Park Ring Road, Leeds LS16 6EB, United Kingdom
+44 (0) 113 278 1708
e-mail: hk@hkeurope.com

United States: Human Kinetics, P.O. Box 5076, Champaign, IL 61825-5076
800-747-4457
e-mail: humank@hkusa.com

Canada: Human Kinetics, 475 Devonshire Road Unit 100, Windsor, ON N8Y 2L5
800-465-7301 (in Canada only)
e-mail: orders@hkcanada.com

Australia: Human Kinetics, 57A Price Avenue, Lower Mitcham, South Australia 5062
08 8277 1555
e-mail: liahka@senet.com.au

New Zealand: Human Kinetics, P.O. Box 105-231, Auckland Central
09-523-3462
e-mail: hkp@ihug.co.nz

This book is dedicated to my former students in high school and college. Thank you for giving me the knowledge to be the best teacher I could be.

Contents

Acknowledgments

Thank you to my family and colleagues who have read, typed, and edited the volumes of pages: Bruce Cartwright, Carrie Dockerty, Barb Hansen, Bill Pitney, Anne Solari, and to the students who took portions of the examination.

Preface

The countdown has begun. You are nearing the end of your college career, and it's time to prepare for passing the National Athletic Trainers' Association (NATA) Board of Certification (BOC) examination. You want to represent your school well and wear the credentials ATC with pride. The big hurdle? Surviving and passing the certification examination.

You probably have several questions. What is on the test? How do I relax while taking the test? How do I register for the test? What are my chances for success? And so on. This manual for preparing for the Athletic Trainers' Certification Examination should answer most if not all of your questions. This manual will also help you review the latest changes and appropriate materials for the certification process. Your basic knowledge and skills in the six domains of athletic training will be assessed.

Over the years, the NATABOC has taken on the task of reviewing and revising the certification process. The certification process has changed to accommodate the many tasks that entry-level athletic trainers must be able to perform. The changes are determined by the Role Delineation Study, which is a job analysis of current practices. As a result of the most recent study, changes have been made in the certification examination. Changes include

- New references
- Curriculum programs for certification
- Single-tasked skill practical
- More practical questions
- Revised domains
- Number of questions per domain

This manual is not intended to replace your four years of athletic training curriculum. Nor is it intended to be used as the sole preparation tool for the certification examination. However, this manual will provide you with valuable insights and strategies for successfully passing the NATABOC certification exam.

The manual is divided into eight chapters. The first two chapters provide all the information you need to put you in the best possible position to pass the test on your first try. In these chapters you'll find useful information about procedures, test structure and administration, and scoring. You'll be apprised of what to expect on test days and given suggestions on what to bring with you to ease the stress of the testing environment. Information on receiving and interpreting your results is included, along with information on what to do when you pass the test—or if you fail. Additionally, helpful hints are provided to improve your studying efficiency.

In chapters 3, 4, and 5 you'll find detailed information about each of the three parts of the examination: the written exam, the practical exam, and the written simulation. For each part of the test, I explain what the test examines, how the test is presented, and the administrative procedures. I also offer several test-taking strategies to help you succeed on test day.

In the final three chapters, I present hundreds of sample study questions designed to make you feel as if you're actually taking the certification examination. The questions are not the exact questions that appear on the test, but they are similar to those you find on each exam. Answering these questions will provide you with an excellent studying opportunity and prepare you to pass the test. These chapters will help you pinpoint weaknesses prior to examination day and will suggest additional resources you can use to strengthen your weaknesses.

Questions for the written and practical examinations appear in the form of multiple choice and Yes or No questions. The written simulation, which tests your decision-making skills in situations a certified athletic trainer faces on a daily basis, provides an opening scenario and asks you to select the best course of action from a list of possibilities. A complete answer key appears in the appendix so you can easily check your answers and assess your ability to pass the test. This material is the most comprehensive list of questions that could possibly appear on a certification examination. The most thorough list of questions currently available for review appears here. There are 600 written multiple choice questions, 38 practical exams, and 20 written simulation tests. Every written question and practical is fully referenced and documented. Because each question is substantiated, you can more easily find and read additional information concerning a subject area, should you choose.

The manual also provides easy-to-understand guidelines for preparing and registering for the test.

The manual for Preparing for the Athletic Trainers' Certification Examination will help you develop strategies for remembering what you learned in college, and doing so under rigorous testing pressure.

To become a certified athletic trainer, you must pass the certification examination. The certification examination is broken down into three main sections: written, practical, and written simulation. This athletic trainer examination review has been designed to assist you and help fill in your areas of weakness in the basic areas of the written examination.

Parts of the written examination are as follows:

A. Prevention

The health care team
Communication
Risks of participation
Rules of sport and techniques
Pre-participation screening
Protective equipment
Conditioning
Anatomical structures
Physiological function
Biomechanics of exercise
Health topics
Social/personal problems
Physics of injury
Safety and sanitation standards
Nutritional practices

B. Recognition, Evaluation, and Assessment

History of injury
Signs and symptoms of injury and illnesses
Metabolic signs and symptoms
Recognition of mechanisms of injury
Psychological signs and symptoms
Effect of improper nutrition
Educating patient via communication
Mechanism of injury
Skills of observation and palpation of injury
Performance of special tests
Patient referral

C. Immediate Care

Emergency techniques in life-threatening situations
Role of prescription drugs in emergency situations
Vital signs
Applying protective devices
First aid

Athletic training procedures
Referral to medical personnel
Educating patient via communication

D. Treatment, Rehabilitation, and Reconditioning

Ongoing evaluation of injury
Anatomical structures
Physiological function
Stages of injury
Restore injured body area
Criteria for return to activity
Nutritional demands of injured athlete
Role of prescription drugs during rehabilitation
Documentation of rehabilitation
Use of modalities
Principles of exercise
Educating patient via communication

E. Organization and Administration

Medical records
Documentation of status
Communication with allied health care providers
Referrals
Documentation of records and distribution of drugs
Policies/procedures
Insurance procedures
Safety and sanitation standards
Budget management

F. Professional Development and Responsibility

Continuing education in all domains
Professional conduct
Law related to athletic training practice
Public relations

The practical portion of the examination will provide 8 to 10 situations for you to demonstrate your care. Usually there are rehabilitation skills, assessment skills, taping, wrapping, and emergency care situations.

The written simulation portion of the examination will present four scenarios. Each scenario asks you to get the athlete through the situation. You are graded on your decision making.

1 CHAPTER

Test Administration

Who could have imagined that, with the invention of sport, today there would be huge stadiums, massive professional salaries, and a whole realm of people who assist athletes to perform better? Athletic trainers became a part of sport almost from the start. Today, athletic trainers practice skills in a multitude of settings including hospitals, schools, colleges, professional sport, industrial, personal training, music halls, and theaters. The skills that athletic trainers have are invaluable to great artists, musicians, actors and actresses, factory workers, athletes, and the general population. Because the skills are so valuable and could possibly cause harm if performed improperly, a need existed to ensure that each athletic trainer obtain a basic level of skills.

The certification examination to become a certified athletic trainer began in the early 1970s. A group of athletic trainers formed a group called the National Athletic Trainers' Association (NATA). The NATA formed a Board of Certification (BOC). The job of the BOC is to generate a test, decide how to administer it, score it, and decide who meets the criteria for passing the test. The BOC was originally a part of the NATA but was separated and incorporated to insure professionalism. The NATA contracts with the BOC to run the certification process for the NATA. The NATA can opt to hire another agency to run the certification examination but thus far has not felt the need to do so. The BOC is made up of 10 certified athletic trainers, who represent each district, and a chairperson. The 10 representatives are elected to their positions within their representative districts (the National Athletic Trainers' Association is divided nationally into 10 districts).

When developing an examination, the key is that the test must be reliable and valid. The definition of "reliable" is that the certification examination must reflect what an athletic trainer does in his work consistently through use of test consistency. For the examination to be "valid," it must be grounded in the principles of athletic training. To determine validity, periodic research is done to determine entry-level skills, which change annually. The research into the skills of the athletic trainer is done via the

Role Delineation Study. The study is sent to a representative cross section of members in the National Athletic Trainers' Association. The members answer questions in each of the six domains regarding the importance and the frequency of each situation or skill addressed. Once members return their questionnaires, the research is compiled to determine the areas of emphasis for an entry-level athletic trainer.

This research is done every few years to ensure the test reflects current practice. The Role Delineation Study was published in 1999 and was a part of the certification test for the first time in 2001.

Once the skills of an entry-level athletic trainer are determined, an exam can be developed. The questions of the examination are written by certified athletic trainers, from commonly used references. Each question must be verified in at least two references. A small group of athletic trainers who specialize in each of the domains scrutinize the questions. The specialized group of athletic trainers must agree that the questions are correct and well written to avoid confusion. Once an examination question is written and approved by the specialized group of athletic trainers, the BOC will put it into the pool of questions available for an actual test. In the written portion of the examination several new questions will be added to an actual examination. These questions are used to determine, from a candidate's perspective, if the question works well or has flaws. If a question has flaws, it may be revised or removed entirely. If the question was determined to work well, it will go into the pool of possible examination questions for the future. Because the test questions are chosen randomly, there might be many questions regarding a single body part, or an area, or none. An examination will not be used again after one year of use.

The history of the certification process has evolved over time. The first certification examination was given in Kansas City and had 150 written questions and an oral practical portion that contained five questions. The oral practical test was administered by three certified athletic trainers. In the early stages of test administration, tests were hand-corrected. Five years ago the certification process underwent an overhaul that resulted in the current examination. Today the certification examination is a three-part test involving a written section, a practical, and a written simulation.

In 1995 the oral practical examination was changed to a practical examination. In the last six years the practical examination has changed from doing multiple skills in one question to a single skill. Today there are between 8 and 10 questions in the practical exam. Each practical question must be found in two references. The examiners involved in the practical exam must be certified athletic trainers, have taken a written test, and have a course on the examination process. The testing of examiners helps to ensure the quality and accuracy of the scoring on the practical. There are three certified athletic trainers in the practical examination, a model, and two examiners. The two examiners for a test are rated on their ability to have corresponding responses to a candidate's skills performed. This is known as "inter-rater reliability." Athletic trainers who score high on the inter-rater reliability, after working a practical exam, are invited back to the next examinations. The day of the practical examination, examiners view a videotape of the practical skills and are told the expectations of each. If you're interested in the examiner training program, call the NATABOC at (877) 262-3926.

The written simulation was added to assure that basic protocols are being used in a variety of basic situations. The written simulation tests decision-making and problem-solving skills. The written simulation was designed to re-create field experiences that can occur in daily athletic training experiences. The written simulation first appeared and was scored in 1987. The written simulation has several sections and averages about 75 items for which to respond. A question in this area is developed to ensure it corresponds to actions and situations in which an entry-level athletic trainer would perform several times in a year. The candidate is asked to choose only items critical to the resolution of the question, at that time, with the information that has been given.

A group of athletic trainers reviews the written simulation questions to determine need for improvement or revision. These questions provide answers that, if selected by a candidate, would cause the situation to worsen. Once a test question is accepted, it is placed into an examination. After an examination, the new question will be viewed for possible problems and revised as needed. The BOC is one of only a few organizations that use this type of testing.

Annually the BOC uses two multiple choice sets of questions, two written simulation sets of questions, and four practical examinations. Some questions may become standards, with a few new experimental questions put in to determine how they work. New tests are placed into use in April of every year.

Most recently the NATA Education Committee has revamped the educational standards. All curriculum programs must meet criteria to have an athletic training curriculum. Since all programs are required to teach the same course work, the standardization of preparation will be achieved. Curriculum programs are reviewed every five years to make sure they continue to meet the requirements.

Required classes include health, human anatomy, physiology, kinesiology, exercise physiology, basic and advanced athletic training, and therapeutic modalities. There must be instructional aids (textbooks, models, audiovisual equipment, team physicians, clinical sites, rehabilitation equipment), and a training room of appropriate size. There must be equal opportunity for all students and strong instructors in all phases of the curriculum. The clinical experience necessary in a curriculum program is 800 hours. Internship programs require 1,500 hours. The clinical hours are required to provide the "hands on" experience that our forefathers used to gain valuable experience through working with injured athletes. Twenty-five percent of clinical hours must be with sport activities such as football, lacrosse, rugby, soccer, gymnastics, wrestling, basketball, hockey, or volleyball, if the candidate is in a curriculum. Internship candidates must have 1,000 hours in a setting where athletics occur (high school, college, or professional sport).

The internship program was designed for colleges or universities that do not meet all the requirements of a curriculum program. The internship program is being phased out and will disappear in January 2004. Those students who are in internship programs must apply for the examination and be eligible by January 2004. No students will be allowed to be in internships after 2001 because the 1,500 hours required for the test cannot be obtained before 2004. Those programs that do not become curriculum programs will no longer be sites for teaching athletic training for the process of certification.

Columbia Assessment Services (CAS) is the agency the BOC uses to ensure a test is valid and reliable. Recently, CAS became a part of CASTLE Worldwide. CAS is responsible for test registration, determining candidate eligibility, correcting the examination, test distribution, ensuring reliability of examiners, ensuring that test questions meet their intent, and getting feedback regarding test questions and policy changes to improve the test and its procedures.

The BOC determines the sites needed for the certification examination. The BOC determines the need for sites and test dates based on the number of candidates in an area and access to the site. There were over 1,000 candidates for tests in 2000. The test sites are supervised by trained individuals called "test site administrators." Test site administrators have the responsibility of organizing the test site by obtaining the certified athletic trainers and models and assigning candidates to the practical examiners. The test site supervisor also determines who will proctor the written exam and written simulation. The test site administrator will explain the examination the day of the test to all the candidates and to the practical examiners. All tests and answer sheets are counted and returned to CAS for processing.

2

CHAPTER

Taking the Test

This chapter helps you prepare for the test by learning everything from how to register for the test to what to expect before, during, and after exam day. Special study hints are also included to help you relax and be as ready as you can be to begin taking your exam.

■ *Who Can Take the Test?*

College graduates or graduation candidates, in their final semester, who can show proof of graduation can take the test. Candidates must complete an application and show proof of course work and requirements necessary to take the certification examination.

■ *Registering for the Test*

Give yourself some lead time to get all your requirements met to take the exam. Candidates who mail in their application and complete their requirements are assigned to test sites on a first-come, first-served basis. Applications must be received by the deadline.

■ *Obtaining an Application*

Tests are given nationwide five times a year and each test date has a deadline for applications to be received. Once you are ready to take the test and have a date and time selected, write or call

NATABOC Administrative Offices
4223 South 143rd Circle
Omaha, NE 68137
Phone: (402) 559-0091

Fax: (402) 561-0598 FAX
www@nataboc.org

To be sure you are registered for exam contact:

Columbia Assessment Services, Inc.
CASTLE Worldwide, Inc.
PO Box 14148
Research Triangle Park, NC 27709-4148
Phone: (919) 572-6880
Fax: (919) 361-2426
www.castlelearning.com

■ *Test Requirements*

After contacting Columbia Assessment Services, Inc., you'll be sent information and the eligibility requirements to take the test. You'll need to gather a lot of information prior to receiving the application so that you are ready when it arrives. Here's what you will need:

1. Names of all colleges and universities you have attended, dates you attended each school, and the name of the degree and the date it was received.

2. The address of a notary public available for notarizing paperwork.

3. For internship students, a copy of the college/university course description for the NATA required classes.

4. The number of hours you have worked in various sports. All hour sheets must be signed and dated by the supervising athletic trainer.

5. The certification number of the sponsoring certified athletic trainer.

6. Your social security number.

7. Date and place you want to take the certification examination, as well as alternative choices in case your first choice is full by the time your application is received. The test is given five times a year, but space is limited. There is no waiting list for sites if you do not get in.

8. A copy of your first aid and cardiopulmonary resuscitation cards or EMT certification. Get a copy, or find your instructor so he can give you a copy of the course record indicating you took and passed the class. If you do not have a copy of the card, you'll need to get a letter from your instructor.

9. Official copies of transcripts from all colleges and universities you have attended.

10. A copy of your NATA student membership card, if you're a member. If you're not a member, taking the test costs more.

11. A check or money order to be sent along with your application. Candidates taking the examination for the first time pay $300. NATA nonmembers may take the test if they meet the criteria and send $350.

12. If you need special accommodations to take the test, you'll need to fill out an Americans With Disabilities Act form, which you can obtain from the NATABOC. The form must be accompanied by medical documentation. (A letter of confirmation will be sent to you once you are assigned to a site. CAS will send you an admission ticket about three weeks before the test.)

13. The address to which you want your results sent.

■ Where Is the Test Held and How Often?

The test is given five times a year at over 100 regional test sites, usually in university or college settings. In 2000, there were 119 test sites around the United States. The test starts at 8 A.M. and goes until noon; it starts again at 1:30 PM and continues until 4:30 PM. You are allowed to leave early if you finish early, but expect the test to be an all-day affair. Don't make plans that force you to rush through the test. If you have come to the test with others, don't rush to finish before or with the others. You will be given time for lunch, but you may want to bring a lunch with you or find your restaurant ahead of time.

■ Changing Your Mind

If you're not ready to take a test you have been assigned to, write the BOC and ask to have a postponement until the next test date. Reach the BOC at 4223 South 143rd Circle, Omaha, NE 68137; phone (402) 559-0091; fax (402) 561-0598; **www@nataboc.org**. There is a refund of 75 percent if you cancel 30 days before the date of the exam, but the request to cancel must be in writing. To reschedule a test, you will need to pay an additional fee of $100. Do not postpone out of fear or anxiety, especially if you know the material. If you have an unusually high anxiety for test taking, you should seek the help of a professional. The proctor and examiners are very aware of the anxiety that can be generated as the result of the test. In the past, special allowances have been made for those who have an unusually high anxiety level, especially during the practical portion of the test. The usual procedure is to allow you to relax and maybe get a drink and come back into the room and proceed where you left off. If you find yourself in this situation, use your visualization and relaxation techniques.

■ *Test Day Procedures*

On the day of the test you will be required to bring your admission ticket, confirmation notification from the BOC, and your driver's license with picture ID. The identification number listed on the admission ticket is required to be on all of your testing materials (answer sheets and cassette for practical). If you arrive late for any portion of the test, you will not be allowed to take that part of the test. You will need to retake that portion of the test and pay an additional fee. All testing sheets for the exam are computerized and require a number two pencil (bring two). The proctor will supply a pencil if you forget. For the written simulation, the marking highlighter pen will be provided. Do not bring any textbooks, coats, backpacks, or paper to the test. The test site is not set up to care for children or visitors. Please make arrangements to accommodate others ahead of time. If you are disruptive during the test, you will be asked to leave and are subject to a retake of the exam and an additional fee.

After you have completed the test, you're not allowed to discuss the content of the exam with anyone. If you're caught doing so you will be put before the BOC review board for disciplinary measures, usually resulting in dismissal (which means you'll never be a certified athletic trainer). One thing good to do after the test is "debriefing," which is simply talking about how you felt during the test, funny little things that happened, how successful you were, and how you're glad it's over. The most common comment from examiners who give the test is, "I remember how I felt after just completing the test." I guess it's a feeling that stays with you the rest of your life.

■ *Helpful Hints*

Preparation is the key to a successful performance on exam day. You can take several steps before and during the test to help you do your best.

Studying for the Exam

Always begin studying in the area that you have the greatest weakness as this will strengthen your confidence in that area, and you will spend the greatest amount of time studying it. As you study the facts, in and around the test, be sure to review the facts daily, as this will strengthen your memorization throughout the process of studying.

Workshops are available for those who want an intensified study program. The ACES workshops are given 10 times a year in locations around the United States. To get more information regarding a workshop, call (757) 221-3407 or visit the Web page at **www.tribeathletics.com/extras/local/sportsmedicine/acesprep.html**. The NATABOC offers a Self-Assessment examination. It can be found on-line at **www.nataboc.org**. The cost is $45. After taking the test, you will receive a report breaking down each domain of the written. This is a good way to focus your learning as the test approaches.

In general, to help you study for the exam I suggest you do the following:

1. Write your goal "to become an ATC." When you drift off or procrastinate, read your goal.
2. Review previous tests from your college career.
3. Become familiar with test directions and formats ahead of time.
4. Understand the point totals for each section of the exam.
5. Read the references recommended in the bibliography of this manual.
6. Don't study while watching television or listening to loud music. Don't sit in a really comfortable chair or you might fall asleep. Eating can also be a distraction.
7. Avoid medication or alcohol that will make you tired or keep you awake (caffeine) just to study. Medications will interrupt the rapid eye movement part of your sleep, and you'll wake up with the feeling that you did not sleep enough. This type of pattern hurts your study time and creates gaps in your memorization of facts.
8. Try to study in a room that simulates the actual site, as this will make you more comfortable on test day.
9. Don't spend time studying an area in which there is disagreement on how to take care of an injury. For example: one textbook might say it's appropriate to apply ice for 40 minutes, while another text says 60. If you run into this kind of discrepancy, get confirmation from several textbooks in the reference list.
10. Items that are done in one section of the country but nowhere else or that are called a particular name should be studied with all the names understood.
11. Remember that thousands of people have passed this test. You can, too.
12. Divide huge domains into smaller categories. This allows you to study smaller segments to reach your goal.
13. Do not wait until the last minute to start studying.
14. If you drift while studying, write down the thought that made you drift so that you don't go back to it until you're done studying.

15. If you're constantly drifting while studying, take a break. Breaks are critical to keep your thought processes going. Take a break that doesn't require you to think much. Now is a good time to load the dishwasher or do laundry.
16. Exercise is essential. Take a break and take care of yourself.
17. Studying for the certification examination is a full-time job. You must study as much as possible. Set up a study schedule and follow your plan.
18. Designate a place to study. Have all your materials within the study area that you need that day.
19. Design flash cards and have someone quiz you.
20. Set study priorities for both daily and weekly goals.
21. Think about what you're learning and give it a real-life application. This will help you remember it later.
22. Look over past exams you have taken in your college courses (generally college exam questions will be more comprehensive than the certification exam).
23. Use a study group to cut down the amount of time you have to spend in any one area. For instance, each group member might be responsible for one section of the body.
24. Use memory joggers to help you remember. For example, a strategy used in medicine is "AMPLE," where A = Allergies, M = Medication, P = Previous medical history, L = Last meal, and E = Events.
25. Include "certified athletic trainer" after your name to help you keep your mind on your goal.
26. Create checklists of tasks to complete. Using the Role Delineation Study and the clinical education competencies will help.
27. Review materials regularly.
28. Study the most difficult material when you're fresh.
29. Reward yourself for completing a task.

Late Start

Okay, so you didn't start studying early enough. Don't panic. Instead, start cramming for the test. Some pointers:

1. Determine the areas to be covered.
2. Get your materials together.

3. Skim chapters, reading only the headings and the areas in the margin. Anything you don't understand after reading the headings, read the paragraph that applies to the heading.
4. Read two quality textbooks and a few textbooks specific to areas of weakness.
5. Vary your areas of study.
6. Emphasize studying areas of weakness.
7. Write things down or highlight a section that is difficult. This way, when you go back to it, the main point will stick out.
8. Review early in the morning the day of the test.
9. Don't scold yourself for getting a late start—that's counter-productive.
10. Repeat the material as many times as you can.

■ *Reducing Anxiety*

Think positively. Do not mull things over with other candidates, as this will raise your anxiety level. If you're concerned about the site or room location, go early. The room used for the written exam may be open if you show up early enough. Sit down in a seat you would normally pick and try it out for comfort. If you don't like it, move! Find a seat where you'll be comfortable for four hours. Keep your shoulders and neck loose. A seat with arms, or a high table, is suitable for this. If you can, try taking a facsimile of a test at that particular site. It's also helpful to get to the testing site at a time similar to when you'll be taking the real test. Try to simulate the test by taking the three sections of the test with the same number of questions and in the same length of time. Notice if the room has any distractions: windows, loud noises, heat or chill, bells, loud clocks, aisle ways, poor lighting, and so on. Students might want to ask the proctor questions in the front of the room. Will this be a distraction for you? You must also decide if your study group will sit together or apart. In some settings, candidates are assigned seats. Try to meet the proctor of the exam while you're there checking out rooms. Walk around in potential practical rooms, too. Again, sit down in a chair and look for distractions.

If you cannot see the site prior to the exam, you may want to spend the night in a hotel close to the site and go over extra early and get a look around. (Staying in a hotel the night before may relieve some of your anxiety about getting lost in an unfamiliar city). Some people have more anxiety being away from home. Decide what is best for you. The NATABOC does keep information on hotels close to each test site if you have an interest.

About one week before the test you should practice some relaxation techniques. You might want to do some deep breathing to help you relax, or some creative visualization. Silently tell yourself, "I will do well, I will relax, I will pass." The technique of creative visualization is very helpful in calming fears. Creative visualization is simply closing your eyes and imagining yourself relaxed and confidently going through the test without any difficulty. Imagine the good feeling upon completion of the test. This is the same technique athletes use to help them through pressure situations. So why shouldn't you use it? Some people believe in a higher power, which they might use to keep emotions in check. If you have a lucky charm, bring it along.

If you have difficulty with sweaty palms during the test, try using a clear spray deodorant. Spray the deodorant on your hands for a week. This will help your hands stay drier during the test. If you sweat profusely, you may want to bring a second set of clothes to change into after lunch or at the end of the examination. You will not be allowed to change during the test. A little anxiety is normal. If you have more than usual, you may want to consult a professional.

■ General Tips for Exam Day

On the night before the test, review areas you think you need to repeat. Lay out all of your clothing, pencils, admission ticket, and lucky charm. Be sure to get a good night's rest. Go to bed early. Do things that relax you: take a hot bath or listen to music. Eat a good meal the night before. Don't drink any caffeine products, as they may keep you awake. Don't take any sleep medications or alcohol that might cause you to oversleep. If you're staying in a hotel, be sure your room is isolated so it will be quiet all night. Consider setting more than one alarm clock to be sure you awake in enough time to get ready and arrive at the test on time.

Clothing

When deciding what to wear for the test, consider something that is comfortable and typical of what you would wear as a certified professional in the training room setting. Khaki pants and a polo shirt are fairly typical. Wearing high heeled shoes or suit coats and ties are outside the realm of comfort, but if you want to, wear them. Do not wear any clothing with your school or team insignia. This has the potential for examiners to treat you in a biased manner. Wear a watch to help you keep track of the time, if you desire.

During the Test

While taking the test, keep your head, neck, and shoulders relaxed. You may wish to rotate your head, neck, and shoulders periodically to keep them loose. Also, take a deep breath and exhale slowly while thinking to yourself, *relax.* Briefly concentrating on something can refocus your attention. Some people press their fingertips together or press their toes into the ground as a way of reducing tension. Do what you can to remain relaxed. Don't focus on what others are doing. Pay attention to what you came to the test for. Your goal is certification.

If you have questions about the examination, ask the proctor. It is the proctor's job to assist you with questions.

■ *Results Notification and Interpretation*

About two weeks after you take the exam, Castle Worldwide will notify you by mail of the results of your test. If you have not heard anything in three weeks, contact Castle Worldwide at (919) 572-6880.

■ *Interpreting Your Score*

When you receive your letter from CAS, your test results will be broken down into three sections: written, practical, and written simulation. You do not have to pass all three sections at the same time. Each section of results will indicate how many points were available, your score, and the passing points needed. The passing point is established by the BOC. The BOC establishes a passing point at which it is believed an athletic trainer is competent to safely service the public. A passing point is established by asking a group of select athletic trainers to determine what the likeliness is that an entry-level candidate will answer this question correctly. An average is then established from the selected group, along with reliability factors for the test. Basically, passing points are based on degree of difficulty of the test as determined by the select group of athletic trainers. The passing point for each section of the test is then set. If a question is changed or removed, the passing point can change. No two tests will likely have the same passing point. You will have to read and compare your score to the passing points needed. If you have the passing points, or more, you have passed that portion. The passing point in this manual is the 70 percentile range for all portions of this examination. The BOC does not use a bell curve to determine passing points, nor is there a number of students who must pass/fail any examination.

General Pass Rates

Based on recent data (Dallas: NATABOC Spring 1993), it appears that candidates who received their college degrees in athletic training score better on the certification test.

■ *Retake Options and Procedures*

You'll be given a score for each section. You can fail all three sections, two sections, or just one section. If you have failed to pass any section of the test, you can ask for a diagnostic report for each section of the test, for which there is a fee. The written portion can be divided by domain to give areas of strengths and weaknesses on the test for a candidate. You may ask that your test score is appealed. Your appeal letter must include reasons you would like your case to be reviewed. You may also ask for a rescoring of the test. All requests must be received within 30 days of results. Candidates are charged a fee for a rescoring of a test. If you failed the practical portion of the test, you can ask that the audio- cassette tape be reviewed if you felt you were badgered but not to determine if a skill was performed properly. If you're treated unfairly during the practical, report to the proctor of the examination. The BOC will notify you of the review of your tests, usually within a month. No test answer sheets or tests are released, as they are confidential.

You must retake within one year any portion of the exam that you have not passed. A retake exam form will be included with your original score notification. You must submit the retake form and fee along with the testing date and site for which you would like to be considered. You must also have current CPR certification at the time of the retake application. If the candidate has failed the exam more than three times, the BOC may recommend additional course work or more hours of supervision before the next retake. If you must retake a single section, the cost is $190. Each additional section retake will cost about $40.

3 CHAPTER

The Written Examination

Test sites determine which portion of the test is done in the morning and afternoon. Lately, the written and practical portions are done in the afternoon. The written examination is designed to examine your ability to remember facts and details. You must be able to relate facts to the specific question asked. Six domains are covered: (1) prevention; (2) recognition, evaluation, and assessment; (3) immediate care; (4) treatment, rehabilitation, and reconditioning; (5) organization and administration; and (6) professional development and responsibility. The answer portion of the test is written in pencil on a computer-generated answer sheet.

Format and Number of Questions

The written examination consists of 150 multiple choice questions, mostly testing your recognition and evaluation abilities, and your management, treatment, and disposition abilities. There will be five possible answers to all multiple choice questions. There are no negatively framed questions in this examination, so do not study that format (for example, "All of the following are correct *except*"). There are no "All of the above" or "only A and B" type answers.

Time Limit

Plan on spending about three hours on the written portion of the exam. If you're working at a fairly rapid pace, no question should take you longer than one minute. This will allow you 30 minutes to review your exam. A test monitor will tell you when to begin and when the test ends. Once you have completed the test and are confident that you are finished, you are allowed to leave the test site.

Scoring

There is only one correct answer to each question, and all questions are worth the same. You'll be penalized for each question you do not complete or answer correctly. This portion of the test is both computer-scored and hand-scored. The hand-scoring is to make sure there are no stray marks from the pencil.

Test-Taking Strategies

Here are some helpful hints for taking the multiple choice test:

- Eliminate incorrect answers to narrow your choices.
- If you draw a blank on a question, as a result of not knowing a word, try to relate it to something else. For example, say you're stuck on the word "mononucleosis." In this case, the stem of the word is *mono,* meaning "one," and *nucleo,* relating to "nucleus."
- If you draw a blank and can't relate anything to the question, skip the question and come back to it later. After you have eliminated incorrect answers, don't be afraid to guess, if necessary.
- After reading a question, first ask yourself for the answer, then look at the possible answers on the test. If the answer you come up with is not one of the choices listed, reread the question.
- Statements that use the terms "always," "never," "all," and "none" are often incorrect, as they leave no room for any exceptions.
- Test writers try to make sure answers are grammatically correct with the stem of the question. For example: When deciding how to match an athlete based on maturity, it is best:

    a. age.
    b. height.
    c. weight.
    d. to use Tanner staging.
    e. skill.

Put your correct answer into the question and read it. Is it grammatically correct? The only correct answer above is "d," as it's the only one that grammatically follows the sentence.

- If you can't eliminate any of the potential answers, consider that writers lean toward answer "b" and "c" more often than any other.

- If you can eliminate a couple of answers but can't get it down to the final one, you have a 50/50 chance, so go ahead and guess.
- If there are sentence-completion questions with a blank space within the sentence, look for an answer that fits the blank. A longer blank means a longer answer and vice versa.
- Try to visualize the page you studied that dealt with the particular question. Visualize yourself reading this page until you get to the information needed to answer the question.
- If you're concerned you'll forget important facts, as soon as the test is handed out write the facts down on the test (not on the desk, as this may be considered cheating). Be sure to erase your notes before handing in the test.
- If you don't recognize a word, or if a word seems out of place, it's a good bet it's an incorrect response.
- When answering questions with numbers in the answer, it's most often a number in the middle.
- Answers longer in detail are often correct. Test writers tend to add quality to correct answers rather than write long-winded decoys.
- Sometimes test writers will write the correct answer in another question of the test. You may want to recall those questions that relate to each other and answer those in combination.

Once you have completed the written test, go back to the questions you skipped and answer them now. Finally, review the entire test and be sure you have not made any errors. You should only change an answer if you know it is wrong or if you read the question incorrectly. Many people change answers when they were correct the first time. Go through your answer sheet and be sure to erase any stray marks. Make sure each answer corresponds to the appropriate question. Don't worry about others finishing before you. Go at your own pace.

4 CHAPTER

Practical Test

You'll be called for the practical portion of the test while you're taking the written exam. When the examiner calls your name, accompany him or her to another room to complete this portion of the test. Feel free to go to the bathroom or get a drink to help you relax from the written portion and mentally prepare to perform the practical.

In the practical testing room you'll find two examiners and a model (the person on whom you'll demonstrate your skills). A candidate's guide will list your questions. You'll be asked to follow along as each of the questions is read to you. Everything that is said in the practical setting is recorded on audiotape. The recording ensures that the examiners read the question properly and that you're treated properly. The tape cannot be reviewed to determine if you have performed a skill.

Once the examiner finishes reading your question, you can reread the question, relax, and think about exactly what is being required of you. The test begins once you begin working on the model. Don't waste your time redoing a skill in an attempt to get more points. Only your first attempt at a skill will be scored.

■ *Format and Number of Questions*

You'll be asked between 8 and 10 questions that allow you to exhibit your skills. The questions cover the first four domains. A few questions might also include taping or wrapping technique, rehabilitation, evaluation, emergency techniques, using a modality, stretching, and general techniques such as skin fold testing, range of motion, Snellen charts, height, and so on.

■ *Time Limit*

Each question's time limit depends on the skill(s) the question is testing. The total test time is designed not to exceed 22 minutes. You'll be given 5 minutes for an evaluation, rehabilitation, and any emergency technique. Any taping or wrapping must be completed in 3 minutes.

Ample time is allotted to allow you to finish all questions. Don't worry that you're able to perform a skill in seconds when you're allowed much more time. Practical tests are designed to accommodate all candidates.

■ Scoring

Points are gained by performing the skill requested. Examiners have sheets that indicate areas that should be covered by specific skills. For example, if the request is a taping technique, the scoring sheet may indicate a task of body part position, skin preparation, application of taping, wrinkle-free tape, and stability of taping technique.

You won't lose a point if you don't complete the taping or wrapping techniques in the allotted time. However, if you have not finished, your score will decrease because you have not completed tasks associated with the skill. You are not given any bonus points for finishing early.

Generally, you won't lose points if you do things out of sequence. However, many emergency techniques must be performed in sequence, so in these cases points are deducted.

Perform each skill that is asked of you. If you have been asked to perform the anterior drawer test, do not perform the Lachmans or pivotal shift test. You'll be scored only on the first test you perform.

■ Test-Taking Strategies

For success during the practical portion of the certification exam, you must be organized. Pre-test preparation is crucial so that you don't exceed the time limits. Learning and practicing the steps in wrapping an ankle, for example, will help you remember them when the heat is on at test time.

Try to anticipate or eliminate possible practical questions. For example, it's unlikely that there will be a performance question on isokinetics, as a machine is too big. Smaller items, such as blood pressure cuffs, are easier to obtain and more likely to be tested.

Remember that the model won't respond verbally to any questions but will follow your directions. There may be questions in which the model will purposely be in the wrong position to ensure that you move him or her into the correct position. The model will not try to circumvent what you're doing but may show things you actually encounter daily. An example is that the model might plantar flex the foot awaiting you to place the foot in neutral for taping. After the foot has been placed in neutral, and you are taping, it is typical for an athlete to lose that neutral, and the model may also do that. Correct the position back to neutral.

When the examiner is reading the question, follow along. If you're a visual learner, follow along in the candidate's guide so that you understand what skill is being asked. If you want to, reread the question. If you are an auditory learner, you may ask the examiner to reread the question a second time. Before proceeding to perform the skill, collect your thoughts and make sure you understand the expectations. Remember that your time does not start until you start performing the skill.

If you forget something along the way and remember as you are performing it, go ahead and show it. Generally, things do not have to be in any particular order. What's most important is to cover the skill thoroughly, do the skill in a tidy fashion, and perform your evaluations bilaterally and at the same time. Failure to do these results in losing points. Talking your way through the skill will not gain you points. You must perform the skill.

Don't forget that the examination begins the minute you walk in the room. What you say, how you act, how you're dressed can influence how an examiner feels when determining if a task was performed correctly. Don't tell examiners what program you're from. Be composed and stay focused. Thank the examiners when you leave.

Written Simulation

The written simulation is the portion that no one will have seen before test day. This portion is designed to indicate how you would deal with real-life decision making using specific scenarios.

■ *Format and Number of Questions*

The written simulation requires that you read a short scenario and then, using the several answers that you're given, select all answers that aid you in the care of the patient. You'll be using a specialized highlighter pen. When selecting an answer you highlight the area that corresponds with the number. The highlighter is dragged horizontally across until a (*) appears, which indicates the end of an answer. Once highlighted, you can read the words that correspond with the answer you have selected. You'll be presented with additional information that may change how you proceed through the scenario. You'll also get feedback on whether your answer was correct. There are four written simulations per examination. Generally, there are five sections to each question and about 75 possible responses.

■ *Time Limit*

You'll have 2.5 hours to complete this section of the test. This test generally is given at 8 o'clock in the morning.

■ *Scoring*

Points are gained by selecting all of the correct answers. Points are deducted for failing to select all of the correct answers and for selecting too many answers (answers that are contraindicated). If you select an answer and halfway through stop so that only a portion of it is highlighted, it will be scored.

Answers in this portion of the test are weighted. Some are worth more than others. Answers are scored on which elements are essential to the scenario. In this portion of the test, those answers that are critically essential are scored with a ++, those essential are scored with a +, neutral answers (those that cause no harm but are not essential) are scored with a 0, those that are contraindicated are scored with a –, and those that are harmful are scored with a – –.

■ *Test-Taking Strategies*

Select answers that expedite the scenario involved. Select only answers that help you in that particular section. Don't jump ahead. Don't select answers out of curiosity or in frustration. Study things in an orderly fashion such as beginning, intermediate, and advanced rehabilitation for each body part.

Ask yourself several questions when taking this portion of the examination:

1. What are the problems?
2. What is the order in which this situation should be resolved?
3. Did an answer change your next move? If so how?
4. What are all the possible outcomes?
5. What will eliminate possible issues?
6. Have I dealt with this problem before? If so, how did I deal with it?
7. What do I need to know to solve this problem?
8. What do I need to do to solve this problem?

Resist the temptation to highlight every answer. Look for connections between answers. After highlighting an answer, ask if it is relevant to the problem. If you make a mistake by highlighting an incorrect response, figure out why you highlighted the wrong response and move on.

6
CHAPTER

Written Examination Questions

There are four complete written exams included in this chapter, with a total of 600 questions. The actual certification test consists of 150 questions. This portion of the text is designed to give you an idea of the types of questions you'll find on the written test. The questions are subdivided into sections on prevention, recognition and evaluation, treatment, rehabilitation, administration and education, and counseling.

A passing point score is listed at the end of each section. The passing point score is 70 percent. Your goal is to score equal to or better than the passing point score. When checking your answers, if you fail to do well in a particular section (e.g., rehabilitation), read the references listed in Appendix A next to those questions missed. This will aid you in your preparation.

■ *Prevention*

Directions: Each of the questions or incomplete statements below is followed by five suggested answers or completions. Select the best answer in each case.

1. **What surface is the best for prevention of injury while running?**
   a. Hills with uneven terrain
   b. Flat, smooth, and somewhat soft
   c. Transverse grade with curves
   d. Rigid and flat
   e. Soft and flat, with a camber
2. **The sole of a shoe can be shock absorbing if it is**
   a. straight lasted.
   b. waffle iron.
   c. stiff heel countered.
   d. flexible forefoot.
   e. cleated.
3. **Tightness of the vastus lateralis or iliotibial tract can lead to**
   a. femoral anteversion.
   b. femoral retroversion.
   c. squinting patellae.

d. patellar tilt or lateral patellar subluxation.
e. pes anserinus bursitis.

4. When reviewing the endurance date from an athlete's isokinetic test of his knee, the first curve is an indication of
a. an artifact.
b. an illiopsoas contraction.
c. a quadriceps contraction.
d. a hamstring contraction.
e. a quadriceps and hamstring contraction.

5. An athlete who has vision of 20/400 is considered
a. normal.
b. farsighted.
c. nonfunctional.
d. color blind.
e. uncorrectable.

6. Body fat norm for an 18-year-old male is
a. 7 percent.
b. 10 percent.
c. 13 to 18 percent.
d. 20 to 24 percent.
e. 25 to 28 percent.

7. When using skin fold calipers on the triceps, to ensure no muscle is pinched
a. do the test at least three times.
b. have the athlete contract the underlying muscle.
c. flex the elbow.
d. abduct the humerus.
e. have the athlete relax.

8. An athlete who has skin boils should
a. avoid participating in strenuous and low-contact sports until resolution.
b. avoid participating in contact and noncontact sports until resolution.
c. avoid participating in contact and limited-contact sports until resolution.
d. avoid participating unless covered then there is no restriction.
e. have no restrictions.

9. Which of the following is considered noncontact?
a. Baseball
b. Gymnastics
c. Volleyball
d. Men's lacrosse
e. Cheerleading

10. Typical systolic blood pressure for an 18-year-old athlete is
a. 80.
b. 100.
c. 120.
d. 130.
e. 160.

11. Typical pulse rate for an 18-year-old athlete is
a. 120.
b. 80.
c. 60.
d. 50.
e. 25.

12. An athlete with one testicle should
a. not play any sports.
b. not play collision sports.
c. not play limited-contact sports.
d. not play noncontact sports.
e. wear a protective cup.

13. **A 20-yard dash during a preparticipation physical determines**
    a. agility.
    b. anaerobic fitness.
    c. aerobic fitness.
    d. endurance.
    e. power.

14. **To prevent dehydration in hot environments athletes should ingest**
    a. 12 ounces of fluid per hour.
    b. 16 ounces of fluid per hour.
    c. 20 ounces of fluid per hour.
    d. 32 ounces of fluid per hour.
    e. 1 to 1.5 liters of fluid per hour.

15. **When humidity is high, the body's ability to dissipate heat**
    a. increases.
    b. decreases.
    c. stays the same.
    d. changes based on metabolism.
    e. changes based on water intake.

16. **The function of the menisci are to**
    a. help absorb shock over a large area.
    b. prevent lateral and medial translation of the joint.
    c. prevent anterior and posterior translation of the joint.
    d. lubricate the joint.
    e. maintain proper alignment of the joint.

17. **Why do varus blows of the knee occur less frequently than valgus?**
    a. Boney structure is more stable.
    b. Ligamentous structure is stronger.
    c. The musculature is stronger.
    d. There are more ligaments laterally.
    e. The other knee protects the medial joint.

18. **Valgus blows of the knee are sustained mainly by**
    a. bones.
    b. ligaments and soft tissue.
    c. menisci.
    d. muscles.
    e. capsule.

19. **When choosing a knee brace for prevention of injuries while playing football, which brace is used for the best protection?**
    a. Stock
    b. Custom-fitted
    c. Neoprene
    d. Durable
    e. Rigid

20. **Normal pulse rate for an adult is**
    a. between 40 and 60.
    b. between 60 and 80.
    c. between 80 and 100.
    d. 100 or more.
    e. below 40.

21. **Which swimmer is most likely to suffer knee pain?**
    a. Backstroker
    b. Freestylers

c. Sidestrokers
d. Butterflyers
e. Breaststrokers

22. The right upper quadrant of the abdomen contains
a. large and small intestine.
b. gallbladder, liver, and large intestine.
c. gallbladder, liver, and pancreas.
d. spleen, liver, and kidney.
e. stomach, spleen, and large intestine.

23. What is the purpose of using ankle braces?
a. To maintain neutral positioning
b. To increase postural control
c. To decrease ankle stability
d. To increase contact with the ground
e. To increase varus stress

24. The definition of obese for men is ____ percent body fat and ____ percent body fat for women.
a. 15, 20
b. 20, 15
c. 20, 40
d. 35, 25
e. 25, 35

25. Dental injuries can almost be eliminated from football using
a. face masks and mouth guards.
b. face masks.
c. mouth guards.
d. gritting teeth just prior to impact.
e. relaxing the jaw just prior to impact.

26. The tarsal tunnel is formed with which muscles?
a. Extensor digitorum and anterior tibialis
b. Peroneus longus and peroneus brevis
c. Tibialis posterior, flexor digitorum longus, and flexor hallucis longus
d. Tibialis posterior and achilles tendon
e. Extensor hallucis longus, extensor digitorum, and posterior tibialis

27. Which test is used to determine power?
a. Treadmill stress test
b. Dips
c. Sit-ups
d. Shuttle run
e. Medicine ball throw

28. Correcting a hamstring imbalance will result in
a. decreased hip pain.
b. greater range of motion in the hip.
c. greater lateral speed.
d. decreased plantar fasciitis injury.
e. decreased hamstring strain and greater vertical jumps.

29. Which person on the health care team should perform goniometric joint measurement during the pre-participation physical?
a. Nurse
b. Medical doctor
c. Student
d. Doctor of osteopathic medicine
e. Athletic trainer

30. In the anatomical position which body part is most lateral?
a. Umbilicus
b. Acromioclavicular joint
c. Thumb
d. Nose
e. Acetabulum

31. Smooth muscle tissue is found in the
a. quadriceps.
b. blood vessels.
c. nerves.
d. heart.
e. aponeuroses.

32. Which nerve cell only sends impulses away from the central nervous system?
a. Neuralgia
b. Ganglia
c. Neuron
d. Motor
e. Sensory

33. What type of joint is the radiocarpal?
a. Hinge
b. Ball and socket
c. Sellar
d. Trochoid
e. Ellipsoid

34. The lubrication fluid of a synovial joint is
a. aqueous.
b. vitreous.
c. synovial.
d. serous.
e. blood.

35. To prevent a football helmet from tilting forward or backward on the head, what type of chin strap is best?
a. Padded
b. A new one
c. A tight one
d. Two-point
e. Four-point

36. The area of skin in which fibers from the spinal cord infiltrate is known as
a. a neuron.
b. parasympathetic nerves.
c. sympathetic nerve.
d. dermatome.
e. reflex arc.

37. To avoid issues resulting from air pollution, practices and games should occur
a. near a fan.
b. during high commuter traffic times.
c. when the temperature is warm.
d. at midday.
e. after the late afternoon.

38. Diastolic pressure is the pressure when the
a. heart is beating.
b. heart is relaxing.
c. heart is about to beat.
d. heart is about to relax.
e. atrioventricular node is firing.

39. To prevent injury in a free-weight room, it is necessary to allow _____ _____ between stations.
a. 6 inches
b. 12 inches
c. 18 inches
d. 2 feet
e. 3 feet

40. **The musculocutaneous nerves innervate the**
    a. anterior muscles of the arm.
    b. posterior muscles of the arm.
    c. anterior forearm.
    d. palm of hand.
    e. posterior of hand.

41. **The radial and ulnar arteries branch immediately from the**
    a. axillary artery.
    b. brachial artery.
    c. subclavian artery.
    d. cephalic.
    e. basilic.

42. **In endurance training bone density will**
    a. increase.
    b. decrease.
    c. no change.
    d. increase at first and then decrease.
    e. decrease at first and then increase.

43. **The sensory dermatome that covers the anterior aspect of the middle three toes and a portion of the anterior skin is**
    a. L2.
    b. L3.
    c. L4.
    d. L5.
    e. Sl.

44. **The angle of Louis lies in the space between the**
    a. first and second ribs.
    b. second and third ribs.
    c. third and fourth ribs.
    d. fourth and fifth ribs.
    e. ninth and tenth ribs.

45. **The sternocleidomastoid muscle provides what action?**
    a. Elevation of the first rib
    b. Depression of the shoulder
    c. Elevation of the clavicle
    d. Flexion of neck toward side of contraction
    e. Extension of neck at lower cervical vertebrae

46. **The proper starting position for the power clean lift is**
    a. head down, hips over the feet, and shoulders slightly forward.
    b. head, shoulders, and hips over the feet.
    c. head and shoulder over the feet and hips behind the feet.
    d. head up, hips and shoulders over the feet.
    e. head up, hips slightly behind feet, and shoulders slightly forward.

47. **A 15 degree rotation of the malleoli to the tibial tubercle is considered**
    a. tibial torsion.
    b. hip anteversion.
    c. hip retroversion.
    d. Legg-Calve Perthes.
    e. slipped capital femoral epiphysis.

48. **Which muscles are responsible for upward rotation of the scapula?**
    a. Teres major and biceps brachii
    b. Deltoid and pectoralis minor

c. Rhomboids and levator scapula
d. Latissimus dorsi and subclavius
e. Trapezium and serratus anterior

49. The recommended maximum normal daily dosage of ibuprofen taken three times daily is
a. 600-1,200 mg after eating food.
b. 600-1,200 mg before eating food.
c. 600-1,800 mg after eating food.
d. 600-2,400 mg after eating food.
e. 200-600 mg after eating food.

50. Which diseases are transmitted via the blood?
a. AIDS and hepatitis
b. Chickenpox and meningitis
c. Rubella and pneumonia
d. Tuberculosis and AIDS
e. Syphilis and mumps

51. The muscles primarily responsible for external rotation of the shoulder include
a. teres major, latissimus dorsi, and subscapularis.
b. anterior deltoid, pectoralis major, and teres minor.
c. posterior deltoid, teres minor, and infraspinatus.
d. trapezium, teres major, and supraspinatus.
e. pectoralis minor, serratus anterior, and posterior deltoid.

52. Ruptures of shoulder muscles are most often due to
a. overuse.
b. trauma.
c. degeneration.
d. varus stress.
e. spontaneous.

53. The most reliable pulse of the lower leg is
a. dorsalis pedis.
b. posterior tibial.
c. anterior tibial.
d. saphenous.
e. deep peroneal.

54. A vegetarian athlete has had previous problems with iron-deficient anemia. What foods would you recommend as good sources of iron?
a. Pork and lamb
b. Cereal and berries
c. Wheat germ and peas
d. Cocoa powder and enriched white bread
e. Nuts and beans

55. The arteries that supply the forearm include
a. axillary.
b. median and radial.
c. basilic.
d. cephalic and median cubital.
e. radial and ulnar.

56. Each pound of weight lost during practice signifies ________ of fluid lost.
a. one gallon
b. one cup
c. one liter
d. one quart
e. one pint

57. When an athlete performs a pull-up with palms supinated, it is easier for the athlete because

a. both triceps and biceps are active.
b. both biceps and brachialis are active.
c. a decreased range of motion occurs at the elbow joint.
d. the shoulder joint is more stable.
e. the coracobrachialis, brachialis, and triceps are active.

58. An athlete with previous plantar fasciitis problems should be encouraged to stretch

a. extensor digitorium brevis and peroneus tertius muscles.
b. gastrocnemius and soleus muscles.
c. the plantar fascia and the anterior tibialis muscle.
d. posterior tibialis and peroneus brevis muscles.
e. flexor hallucis longus and plantaris muscles.

59. Which of the following is a social aspect of preventing stress?

a. Relaxation
b. Imagery
c. Friends
d. Massage
e. Goal setting

60. Fingers have what movements?

a. Flexion and extension
b. Flexion, extension, adduction, and abduction
c. Flexion, extension, adduction, abduction, and circumduction
d. Flexion, hyperextension, adduction, and abduction
e. Pronation, supination, flexion, and extension

61. The thumb is capable of what movement that fingers cannot perform?

a. Flexion
b. Extension
c. Adduction
d. Hyperextension
e. Opposition

62. The appearance of a faun's beard is indicative of

a. lordosis.
b. kyphosis.
c. high levels of testosterone.
d. growth spurt.
e. bony defect.

63. An athlete in need of losing weight over a short span of time can accomplish this through rapid weight loss. The weight loss will most likely result from

a. muscle loss.
b. fat loss.
c. bone loss.
d. connective tissue loss.
e. fluid loss.

64. The primary movement created by flexor carpi radialis is

a. pronation of the forearm.
b. flexion of the wrist.

c. extension of the fingers.
d. abduction of the thumb.
e. flexion of the first phalanx.

65. The radial nerve is more often injured when there is a fracture of the
a. proximal one third of the humerus.
b. distal one third of the humerus.
c. proximal one third of the radius.
d. distal one third of the radius.
e. head of the humerus.

66. Which segment of blood is responsible for releasing chemicals that form blood clots?
a. Leukocytes
b. Erythrocytes
c. Platelets
d. Plasma
e. Histamines

67. For one pound of fat loss to occur, how many kilocalories must be expended?
a. 2,400
b. 2,800
c. 3,200
d. 3,500
e. 5,000

68. To prevent spinal injuries in ice hockey, rules are enforced to
a. prevent checking from behind.
b. prevent checking below the waist.
c. make sure neck and throat guards are worn.
d. make sure mouth guards are worn.
e. make sure mouth guards, throat guards, and full face masks are worn.

69. Which digit of the hand contains sesamoids?
a. First
b. Second
c. Third
d. Fourth
e. Fifth

70. The Food and Drug Administration requires what minimal information on the prescription label of medications?
a. Drug name, date of dispensing, patient name, quantity, instruction for use, name of physician, and intended use
b. Drug name, date of dispensing, patient name, quantity, and instruction for use
c. Date of dispensing, patient name, quantity, instruction for use, and name of physician
d. Patient name, quantity, instruction for use
e. Drug name, date of dispensing, patient name, quantity, side effects, contraindications, warnings, name of pharmacy, and instruction for use

71. Which muscle can be controlled both voluntarily and involuntarily?
  a. Heart
  b. Pupil
  c. Diaphragm
  d. Intestines
  e. Biceps

72. Which of the following are risk factors that are controllable when preventing heart disease?
  a. Age
  b. Gender
  c. Heredity
  d. High blood pressure
  e. Ethnicity

73. Which of the following ways provides the rescuer protection prior to infectious transmission?
  a. Covering his mouth when he coughs or sneezes, and then working on an athlete
  b. Washing hands before working on an athlete and re-using gloves
  c. Using others' clothing and combs
  d. Two-way valve pocket mask and mouth-to-mouth breathing
  e. One-way valve pocket mask and gloves

74. When a person breathes, physics dictates that as
  a. pressure increases, volume increases.
  b. pressure increases, volume equalizes.
  c. volume decreases, pressure equalizes.
  d. volume increases, pressure decreases.
  e. volume increases, pressure increases.

75. The most prominent spinous process of the cervical vertebrae is
  a. C3.
  b. C4.
  c. C5.
  d. C6.
  e. C7.

76. The best indicator of the fitness of the cardiorespiratory system is
  a. resting heart rate.
  b. maximal oxygen consumption ($\dot{V}O_2$ max).
  c. residual volume.
  d. Krebs cycle efficiency.
  e. rate of recovery from exercise.

77. To create greater space between lumbar vertebrae
  a. extend the spine.
  b. flex the spine.
  c. hyperextend the spine.
  d. lateral flex and extend the spine.
  e. rotate the spine.

78. Which physiological adaptation increased with both resistance and aerobic training?
  a. Capillary density
  b. Body fat
  c. Creatine phosphokinase activity
  d. Vertical jump ability
  e. Mitochondrial density

79. Posterior lateral disk protrusions are most often in
a. cervical.
b. thoracic.
c. lumbar.
d. cervical and lumbar.
e. thoracic and lumbar.

80. Warning signs of low weight disordered eating include
a. hiding food and eating more than three times per day.
b. use of diet pills and neglecting family.
c. spending excessive time in front of a mirror and not able to stop eating.
d. low self-esteem and eating alone.
e. excessive weight gain and memory loss.

81. Spotting is not necessary for which form of resistance training?
a. Overhead exercises
b. Over-the-face exercises
c. Dumbbell exercises
d. Power exercises
e. Lunges

82. Exercise adaptations that are greater physiological changes in men than those in women include
a. improved respiratory changes.
b. muscle girth and fat-free mass.
c. increased percent max $\dot{V}O_2$.
d. improved cardiac changes.
e. decreased resting heart rate.

83. To prevent back injuries while lifting, a person should
a. keep back straight, crouch, and place object on the back.
b. keep feet spread wider than shoulder-width apart.
c. keep feet together.
d. crouch, keep back straight, and let legs do the lifting.
e. make sure shoulders and hips are rotated in opposite directions.

84. What nutritional need will fulfill an athletes' physiological need to increase length of time in competition?
a. Protein
b. Water
c. Carbohydrates
d. Vitamins
e. Minerals

85. When breathing stops brain damage occurs
a. as soon as breathing stops.
b. after 2 minutes.
c. between 4 and 6 minutes.
d. at 8 minutes.
e. at 10 minutes.

86. The American Medical Association recommends the employment of a certified athletic trainer in what setting?
a. Recreational sports
b. Secondary schools
c. Collegiate level
d. Sports medicine clinics
e. Professional sports

87. The portion of the heart that pumps blood to the lungs is
a. aorta.
b. right atrium.
c. left atrium.
d. right ventricle.
e. left ventricle.

88. As an athletic trainer, you are in need of information regarding conditioning, nutrition, and body composition. Which health care professional best fulfills the aforementioned needs?
a. Nutritionist
b. Biomechanist
c. Exercise physiologist
d. Strength and conditioning coach
e. Nurse

89. The pelvis contains two cavities formed by the
a. ilium, ischium, and pubis.
b. ilium and sacrum and the pubis, ischia, and coccyx.
c. upper ilium and the sacrum, pubis, ischia, and lower ilium.
d. large and small intestine and the bladder.
e. sacrum, coccyx, and pubis.

90. Defective electrical equipment in the training room should be
a. tested annually.
b. tested bi-annually.
c. tested immediately.
d. removed from the facility immediately.
e. grounded.

91. Weightlifting belts should be used
a. when lifting anything overhead.
b. if the athlete has lordotic posture.
c. when power lifting.
d. for near-maximal or maximal efforts that stress the back, or whenever the athlete chooses.
e. for lunges, dead lifts, and clean and jerks.

92. What percent of oxygen is in the air a person exhales?
a. 5
b. 16
c. 21
d. 100
e. 760

■ Recognition, Evaluation, and Assessment

Directions: Each of the questions or incomplete statements here is followed by five suggested answers or completions. Select the best answer in each case.

93. Which organ refers pain to the right side of the neck?
a. Liver
b. Spleen
c. Brain
d. Lungs
e. Gallbladder

94. Compression upon the long axis of the femur is used to
a. relax muscle tissue.
b. decrease swelling.

c. determine a fracture of femur.
d. increase circulation.
e. determine Legg-Calve Perthes.

95. **When testing cranial nerve I it can be done by**
a. having the athlete move eyes.
b. having the athlete talk.
c. having the athlete balance.
d. having the athlete smell a strong odor.
e. shrug his shoulders.

96. **Testing cranial nerve VII is accomplished by**
a. having the athlete close eyes and mouth.
b. having the athlete look laterally.
c. having the athlete swallow.
d. having the athlete stick his tongue out.
e. having the athlete read a chart.

97. **A positive Romberg test is an indication of a**
a. shoulder injury.
b. cerebral injury.
c. spleen injury.
d. appendix infection.
e. retinal injury.

98. **The Valsalva maneuver, if positive, is an indication of**
a. brain injury.
b. lordosis.
c. herniated disk.
d. spondylolysis.
e. spondylolisthesis.

99. **For the purpose of communication, when an athlete is talking about a new injury or illness, the athletic trainer should**
a. write everything down.
b. repeat everything back to the athlete to check correctness.
c. have another person record the conversation.
d. keep eye contact and listen with intent.
e. interrupt to clarify.

100. **When performing Speed's test the examiner must palpate the**
a. humerus near the bicipital groove.
b. occipital area of the skull.
c. ischial tuberosity.
d. lateral aspect of the knee.
e. calcaneous.

101. **An athlete with genu recurvatum can be compensating for**
a. rectus femoris weakness.
b. lordosis.
c. scoliosis.
d. weak posterior thoracic musculature.
e. patellofemoral tracking problems.

102. **Clawhand results from injury to the**
a. median and ulnar nerves.
b. radial nerve.
c. blood supply.
d. muscles.
e. muscles, nerves, and blood supply.

103. An athlete comes to you with a new injury. What historical questions need to be asked before observation, palpation, and special tests are performed?

a. Open-ended questions
b. Primary complaint, cause, pain referral points, time of day injury occurred, type of surface injury occurred upon, and weather conditions
c. Primary complaint, cause of injury, extent of disability, previous injuries to area, and family history of same or similar injuries
d. Primary complaint, cause of injury, extent of disability, and previous injuries to area
e. Primary complaint, cause of injury, and extent of disability

104. Hallux rigidus can result from

a. fracture of intra-articular surface.
b. improper mechanics.
c. improperly fitted shoes.
d. heredity.
e. pes cavus.

105. Sulcus sign is an indication of instability of the

a. patella.
b. hip.
c. knee.
d. shoulder girdle.
e. shoulder joint.

106. A Colles' fracture involves the

a. radius and ulna.
b. radius.
c. talus.
d. calcaneus.
e. metatarsal.

107. A flexible scoliosis will

a. disappear with hyper-extension of the back.
b. disappear in a prone position.
c. disappear with lateral bending.
d. appear when lateral bending to the dominant side.
e. appear when lateral bending away from the dominant side.

108. You've determined that an athlete is a malingerer. This is the third time this athlete has been assessed this way. What are the most likely causes of a repeat malingerer?

a. Lack of playing time and pressure from family members
b. Trying to get money for insurance and obtaining goals
c. Loss of starting position and desire to work in the training room
d. Desire to make people happy and lack of desire to play
e. Fear and need for attention

109. A right-handed golfer reports pain over the medial epicondyle of the right

elbow. What is the likely cause of this epicondylitis?
a. Throwing a club
b. Carrying the bag of clubs
c. Pronating on the follow-through
d. Having too small of a grip
e. Hitting the ground with the club

110. The stages of reaction to an injury include
a. shock, denial, anger, depression, and acceptance.
b. denial, anger, bargaining, and adaptation.
c. denial, anger, bargaining, and depression.
d. crisis, shock, post-traumatic stress, adaptation, and resolution.
e. disbelief, depression, post-traumatic stress, and resolution.

111. Lateral epicondylitis can be determined using
a. active resistive motion with the athlete trying to pronate, extend, and radial deviate the wrist.
b. passive motion with the athlete trying to pronate, extend, and radial deviate the wrist.
c. active motion with the athlete trying to pronate, extend, and radial deviate the wrist.
d. active resistive motion with athlete trying to supinate, extend, and ulnar deviate the wrist.
e. passive motion with the athlete trying to supinate, extend, and ulnar deviate the wrist.

112. Varus stress test of the elbow is used to determine
a. lateral collateral ligament.
b. medial collateral ligament.
c. biceps tendon insertion.
d. ulnar nerve function.
e. pronator teres muscle.

113. A positive pinch test is an indication of
a. radial nerve injury.
b. interossei nerve injury.
c. ulnar nerve injury.
d. adductor pollicis muscle injury.
e. flexor digitorum profundus and adductor pollicis muscle injury.

114. Finkelstein test is used to determine a
a. wrist fracture.
b. range of motion of the wrist.
c. sprain of the thumb.
d. carpal tunnel syndrome.
e. de Quervain's disease.

115. Which nerve is impaired when there is a positive Phalen's test?
a. Sciatic
b. Superior gluteal
c. Ulnar
d. Median
e. Radial

116. When facial hair re-enters the skin, causing pus, it creates
a. furuncle.
b. folliculitis.

c. scabies.
d. dermatitis.
e. eczema.

117. An athlete has had difficulty returning to participation because of flashbacks of an old injury. This is a sign of
a. denial.
b. post-traumatic stress disorder.
c. clinical depression.
d. suicidal tendencies.
e. malingering.

118. During the Valsalva maneuver, the examiner needs to be prepared for the athlete to
a. vomit.
b. bleed.
c. get dizzy.
d. cry.
e. have difficulty breathing.

119. How would the athletic trainer know if an athlete is faking a sciatic nerve injury?
a. Have the athlete walk
b. Have the athlete jump
c. Apply electrical stimulation to the nerve
d. Have the athlete perform the Stork test
e. Have the athlete perform the Hoover test

120. The Kernig/Brudzinski test is performed while the athlete is in what position?
a. Standing on both legs
b. Standing on one leg
c. Seated
d. Lying supine
e. Lying prone

121. The straight leg raise test is used to determine
a. hip flexion.
b. hip extension.
c. hamstring tightness.
d. sacroiliac problems.
e. injury of the gluteus medius muscle.

122. The primary difference between a posterior hip dislocation and hip fracture is
a. increased pain with hip fracture.
b. inability to move a hip dislocation.
c. there is numbness with a hip dislocation.
d. inability to straighten the hip dislocation.
e. hip fracture causes external rotation and hip dislocation causes internal rotation.

123. The Thomas test is used when the athletic trainer suspects
a. sciatica.
b. iliopsoas tightness.
c. weak abdominal musculature.
d. herniated disk.
e. adductor weakness.

124. The cause of periodontitis is
a. trauma to the eye.
b. bacterial infection.
c. faulty alignment.
d. eating high amounts of carbohydrates.
e. lack of dental hygiene.

125. When performing the Patrick's/Faber test the leg is
   a. flexed.
   b. extended.
   c. abducted and externally rotated.
   d. abducted and internally rotated.
   e. adducted and internally rotated.

126. To check for a tight tensor fascia latae the examiner may use
   a. Trendelenburg test.
   b. Nobles test.
   c. Patrick's test.
   d. Ober test.
   e. Thomas test.

127. Contributing factors that may result in medial tibial stress syndrome include
   a. running in the same direction daily and pes planus.
   b. excessive stretching and hard running surface.
   c. muscle fatigue and overuse.
   d. excessive contraction and faulty running gait.
   e. excessive change of direction and excessive toe flexion.

128. A true leg-length discrepancy is measure by which points?
   a. Anterior superior iliac spine and medial malleolus
   b. Anterior superior iliac spine and lateral malleolus
   c. Pubis and calcaneous
   d. Femoral head and lateral malleolus
   e. Patella and medial malleolus

129. Which of the following questions is open-ended to allow the athlete to describe an injury?
   a. Is this like last time?
   b. Did you get the number of the guy who hurt you?
   c. Where does it hurt?
   d. Does it hurt over your ACL?
   e. The spot for your pain is right here. Correct?

130. Intervertebral disc herniation of the cervical spine occurs most often between which vertebrae?
   a. C2 and C3
   b. C3 and C4
   c. C4 and C5
   d. C5 and C6
   e. C6 and C7

131. The Nobles test is used to determine
   a. patellar tendinitis.
   b. bursitis.
   c. lateral meniscus injury.
   d. illiotibial band friction.
   e. abductor strain.

132. The most common mechanism of injury for meniscus is
   a. blow to lateral aspect of knee.
   b. blow to medial aspect of knee.
   c. foot planted with trunk rotation.

d. rotation of knee.
e. alignment problems.

133. To properly test for posterior sag, the knee position is
a. flexed to 90 degrees.
b. flexed to 60 degrees.
c. flexed to 30 degrees.
d. flexed to 30 degrees and then fully extended.
e. fully extended.

134. A low back muscle strain will create pain with what movements?
a. All movement
b. Active flexion
c. Passive flexion and active extension
d. Lateral flexion
e. Passive extension

135. What area of the bone of an adolescent is the weak area of the bone?
a. Head
b. Neck
c. Mid-shaft
d. Distal shaft
e. Apophysis

136. The Slocum test when performed with internal rotation if positive is an indication of
a. illiotibial friction.
b. patellar subluxation.
c. posterior cruciate injury.
d. anterolateral rotary instability.
e. anteromedial rotary instability.

137. An athlete whose diet consists of excessive amounts of vitamin C will likely experience
a. nerve impairment.
b. increased bleeding time.
c. dry skin.
d. diarrhea.
e. headaches.

138. The Spurling test is used to evaluate
a. neck strains.
b. cervical spine compression pathology.
c. sciatica.
d. shoulder impingement.
e. subluxation of bicipital tendon.

139. Deceleration with a cutting motion is likely to lead to which knee injury?
a. Anterior cruciate
b. Posterior cruciate
c. Medial meniscus
d. Medial collateral
e. Lateral collateral

140. To determine if there is an injury to the lateral collateral ligament perform the
a. Hughston's test.
b. Apley's distraction test.
c. varus stress test.
d. valgus stress test.
e. Slocum test.

141. An injury to the volar plate that causes flexion of the proximal interphalangeal joint and extension of the distal interphalangeal joint is known as
a. mallet finger.
b. jersey finger.
c. boutonniere deformity.
d. pseudo-boutonniere deformity.
e. Bennett's fracture.

142. Apley's distraction test when positive indicates
a. subluxation.
b. ligament injury.
c. medial meniscus injury.
d. lateral meniscus injury.
e. circulatory.

143. An anterior talofibular ligament sprain can be determined using the
a. talar tilt test.
b. percussion test.
c. medial stress test.
d. posterior drawer test.
e. anterior drawer test.

144. The starting position of the ankle when performing the talar tilt test is
a. dorsiflexion.
b. plantarflexion.
c. joint neutral.
d. inversion.
e. eversion.

145. To perform the percussion test properly the foot is
a. dorsiflexed.
b. plantar flexed.
c. joint neutral.
d. inversion.
e. eversion.

146. Possible popliteal tendinitis is assessed using what?
a. Varus stress test
b. McMurray test
c. Straight leg dorsi flexion test
d. Ober test
e. Figure 4 position

147. Pes cavus is often associated with which toe condition?
a. Corns
b. Morton's toe
c. Claw toes
d. Hammer toe
e. Ingrown toenails

148. The mechanism of injury for a posterior cruciate includes
a. rotation and varus stress.
b. hyperflexion and shearing.
c. torsion and valgus stress
d. hyperextension and direct impact to the anterior tibia.
e. direct impact to the posterior tibia and heredity.

149. An athlete complains of severe headaches, dry cough, diarrhea, weight loss, night sweats, and unexplained blotches under the skin. What illness do you suspect?
a. HIV
b. Migraine headache
c. Sickle cell anemia
d. Hepatitis
e. Chicken pox

150. An amenorrheic athlete may exhibit symptoms of
a. painful menstruation, increased bone density, and regular menstrual cycles.
b. bone loss, absence of menstrual cycle, increased exercise, and decreased estrogen.
c. low levels of exercise, high food intake, high estrogen levels, and painful menstruation.

d. nausea, bloating, breast tenderness, and absence of menstrual cycle.
e. inability to become pregnant, low bone density, increased exercise, and increased estrogen.

151. A field hockey player reports that she is "too fat." Upon inquiry she says that she does not binge or purge, but she rarely eats. What do you suspect?
a. Gastroenteritis
b. Bulimia nervosa
c. Indigestion
d. Anorexia nervosa
e. Pancreatitis

152. A basketball player has a positive McBurney's point. What illness or injury do you suspect?
a. Liver contusion
b. Ruptured bladder
c. Ruptured spleen
d. Appendicitis
e. Kidney contusion

153. An athlete has indicated on his physical he has exercise-induced asthma. What are the signs and symptoms you need to be concerned with for early recognition of this situation?
a. Chest tightness, wheezing, coughing, shortness of breath just after exercise
b. Facial pain, nasal discharge, coughing just after exercise
c. Headache, tearing, shortness of breath, and chest pain
d. Wheezing, productive cough, and sneezing
e. Radiating pain into left shoulder, chest tightness, and coughing

154. Bronchitis is indicated by
a. sneezing, difficulty swallowing, and hoarseness.
b. malaise, sneezing, coughing, and headache.
c. productive cough and wheezing.
d. hoarseness, fatigue, and wheezing.
e. fever, enlarged lymph nodes, and sore throat.

155. A cross country runner complains of pain on the pubic synthesis and the inability to run. The athletic trainer should suspect
a. bladder infection.
b. hernia.
c. leg length discrepancy.
d. osteitis pubis.
e. Legg-Calve Perthes.

156. Chlamydia in males is distinguished from other sexually transmitted diseases by
a. watery discharge from the penis, groin pain, and fever.
b. mild itching and painful urination.
c. white discharge from the penis.
d. thick yellow or green discharge from the penis.
e. no symptoms.

157. Lack of exercise, laxative abuse, lack of fiber, or emotional distress are common signs and symptoms of
a. hemorrhoids.
b. diarrhea.
c. gastroenteritis.
d. colitis.
e. constipation.

158. The common cold is characterized by
a. fever, productive coughing, shortness of breath.
b. malaise, clear nasal discharge, chills, and fever.
c. sore throat, malaise, enlarged lymph glands, and coughing.
d. dizzy spells, inner ear infection, coughing, and malaise.
e. sneezing, nasal discharge, and tearing.

159. An athlete who has a bright red conjunctiva, along with itching and watering of the eye, is likely suffering from
a. conjunctivitis.
b. subconjunctival hemorrhage.
c. detached retina.
d. corneal abrasion.
e. sty.

160. A cross country athlete is unconscious and has a fruity breath smell. Prior to becoming unconscious his running partner indicates the athlete was complaining of thirst, abdominal pain, and confusion. The athlete progressively becomes more ill over time. These symptoms cause you to conclude the athlete is
a. an alcoholic.
b. in a diabetic coma.
c. in diabetic shock.
d. hypothermic.
e. hyperthermic.

161. Dysmenorrhea is indicated by what symptoms?
a. Painful urination
b. Absence of menstruation
c. Infrequent menstrual cycles
d. Painful defecation
e. Abdominal pain

162. An athlete who has skin vesicular eruptions on his trunk and inside his mouth has symptoms of
a. chicken pox.
b. syphilis.
c. measles.
d. German measles.
e. mumps.

163. A diet deficient in copper will result in
a. anemia.
b. limb length growth problems.
c. greater tooth decay.
d. osteoporosis.
e. lack of energy.

164. A diet with an excess of calcium will result in
a. kidney stones.
b. calcium deposits in soft tissues.
c. hypertension.

d. heart problems.
e. gastritis.

165. Signs and symptoms of gastroenteritis include
a. belching, vomiting, and flatulence.
b. constipation, flatulence, and abdominal cramping.
c. nausea, indigestion, flatulence, and diarrhea.
d. constipation, vomiting, and abdominal cramping.
e. diarrhea, rectal bleeding, and vomiting.

166. A common sign or symptom of gonorrhea in females is
a. a white vaginal discharge.
b. a green or yellowish vaginal discharge.
c. painful urination.
d. vaginal itching.
e. yeast-like discharge.

167. The ischiofemoral ligament functions to
a. assist with abduction.
b. assist with rotation.
c. prevent hyperflexion.
d. prevent hyperextension.
e. hold the femoral head in acetabulum during extension.

168. Women distance runners who are amenorrhic are prone to
a. fractures.
b. plantar fasciitis.
c. abdominal pain.
d. low back pain.
e. proteinurea.

169. Hypoglycemia in an athlete can occur as a consequence of
a. eating too much food.
b. too much exercise.
c. diarrhea.
d. vomiting.
e. too little insulin.

170. A rapid, strong pulse is indicative of what heat-related issue?
a. Heat exhaustion
b. Heat stroke
c. Heat cramps
d. Heat stress
e. Hypothermia

171. Oligomenorrhea has a pattern of
a. long cycles.
b. short cycles.
c. painful cycles.
d. no cycles.
e. regular cycles.

172. Metabolic shock can occur with uncontrolled
a. diarrhea.
b. blood loss.
c. infection.
d. asthma attack.
e. epileptic seizure.

173. Which of the following aids in the process of blood clotting?
a. Vitamins A and D
b. Aloe and Vitamin E
c. Vitamin B_{12} and zinc
d. Vitamin K and calcium
e. Potassium and magnesium

174. What ethnic group is more likely to have hypertension?
a. Asian
b. Caucasian
c. American Indian
d. Hispanic
e. African-American

175. A typical reading for high blood pressure is
   a. 120/80 mmHg.
   b. 90/80 mmHg.
   c. 100 mm Hg systolic or 180 mm Hg diastolic.
   d. 140 mm Hg systolic or 90 mm Hg diastolic.
   e. 180 mm Hg systolic or 60 mm Hg diastolic.

176. Which organs are likely affected during a sickle-cell crisis?
   a. Stomach, lungs, brain, and spleen
   b. Liver, heart, pancreas, and intestines
   c. Heart, lungs, liver, and gallbladder
   d. Spleen, kidneys, lungs, and heart
   e. Central nervous system, pancreas, stomach, and heart

177. An athlete who has sickle-cell anemia is more likely to have an attack if
   a. he is at high altitudes of 2,500 feet above sea level or more.
   b. he eats high amounts of red meat.
   c. the air is dry.
   d. the weather is cold while exercising.
   e. he is exercising and resting every half hour.

178. Which viral illness with a cough may progress into bronchitis?
   a. Hay fever
   b. Common cold
   c. Pharyngitis
   d. Laryngitis
   e. Influenza

179. A quarterback has a sore throat, malaise, enlarged tonsils, a fever, enlarged lymph nodes, and an enlarged spleen. What illness or disease is suspected?
   a. Hepatitis
   b. Infectious mononucleosis
   c. Common cold
   d. Leukemia
   e. AIDS

180. Hyperventilation is differentiated from other respiratory distresses by
   a. relief from additional oxygen intake.
   b. tracheal deviation.
   c. wheezing.
   d. crackling sensation under the skin about the upper thorax.
   e. numbness of the lips and dizziness.

181. The three primary causes of shock are
   a. dehydration, spinal cord injury, and femur fracture.
   b. decreased blood pressure, rapid pulse, and vomiting.
   c. organ failure, increased blood pressure, and lack of oxygen.
   d. central nervous system failure, vessel constriction, and decreased oxygen capacity.
   e. pump failure, volume loss, or vessel dilation.

182. **Some primary signs of shock include**
   a. nausea, thirst, dizziness, and anxiety.
   b. fainting, seizures, cyanosis, and dilated pupils.
   c. vomiting, sweating, cold skin, and rapid weak pulse.
   d. fractures, internal injuries, bee sting, and heart attack.
   e. irregular breathing, constricted pupils, anxiety, and dizziness.

183. **An injured athlete should be referred for counseling if she shows signs of**
   a. grief.
   b. substance abuse.
   c. a sexual disorder.
   d. compulsion for food.
   e. neurosis.

184. **Syncope may result from**
   a. cardiac failure.
   b. stitch in the side.
   c. alcohol intoxication.
   d. cystitis.
   e. sickle-cell anemia.

185. **An athlete tests positive for cocaine. He indicates he has not used the drug in a month. What should the athletic trainer do?**
   a. Refer for counseling and assessment.
   b. Do nothing.
   c. Apologize for the false accusation.
   d. Document and watch for corroboration.
   e. Search the Athlete's locker.

186. **Severe cases of acne vulgaris appear on which body parts?**
   a. Buttocks
   b. Neck
   c. Lower back
   d. Lower extremities
   e. Abdomen

187. **Acne vulgaris becomes more irritated by**
   a. bacteria.
   b. a virus.
   c. cool weather.
   d. dry air.
   e. astringent lotions.

188. **A hair follicle with a fluctuant mass that is tender is known as**
   a. cellulitis.
   b. acne vulgarism
   c. eczema.
   d. furuncle.
   e. contact dermatitis.

189. **Pneumonia is an infection of the**
   a. trachea.
   b. alveoli.
   c. bronchi.
   d. esophagus.
   e. vocal cords.

190. **Rales are commonly heard when an athlete has**
   a. pneumonia.
   b. influenza.
   c. bronchitis.
   d. ear infection.
   e. peritonitis.

191. **Gastritis is aggravated by**
   a. milk and exercise.
   b. aspirin and alcohol.
   c. relaxation and aluminum hydroxide.

d. vomiting and magnesium.
e. cigarette smoking and cold weather.

192. Diarrhea that continues for several days can result in
a. vomiting.
b. colitis.
c. gastritis.
d. dehydration.
e. hemorrhoids.

193. With a spinal fracture of the tibia caused by rotation, the force is known as
a. torsion.
b. strain.
c. compression.
d. pull.
e. sheer.

194. A potentially fatal disease that causes muscle spasms, rigidity, and eventually death from asphyxiation, is known as
a. heat stroke.
b. heat exhaustion.
c. heat cramps.
d. third-degree concussion.
e. tetanus.

195. A positive piano key sign is an indication of
a. shoulder dislocation.
b. injury of the coraco-clavicular ligaments.
c. fracture of clavicle.
d. tear of posterior cruciate.
e. ankle dislocation.

196. Death from hypothermia will occur about two hours after
a. unconsciousness.
b. being outdoors.
c. shivering starts.
d. frostbite.
e. decreased pulse rate.

197. An athlete presents with pain in the upper back and abdomen. What disease do you suspect?
a. appendicitis
b. pancreatitis
c. pelvic inflammation
d. kidney stones
e. diverticulitis

198. Scabies is distinguished from other skin infections by
a. scaling, redness, and fever.
b. itching, skin elevation, and microscopic viewing of mite.
c. itching, skin elevation, and microscopic viewing of crab.
d. itching, scaling, and fissures.
e. circular yellow scaling, swelling, and blistering.

199. A knee joint that has untreated ligamentous instability is likely to cause
a. chondromalacia.
b. fractures.
c. bursitis.
d. tendinitis.
e. osteoarthritis.

200. Biomechanical bone strength is influenced by
a. load rate, load direction, and muscle activity.
b. elastic deformation and ligament stability.
c. genetics and strain.
d. bone type and shear forces.
e. nutrition and stiffness.

201. Abnormal loading of the tibia, combined with high compression, can lead to
a. an oblique fracture.
b. a spiral fracture.
c. a comminuted fracture.
d. a greenstick fracture.
e. an osteochondral fracture.

202. The athletic trainer can differentiate between deep and superficial somatic pain by
a. the athlete telling the athletic trainer.
b. deep being longer lasting and related to bones, muscles, or joints.
c. deep being periodically painful.
d. biofeedback.
e. hypnosis.

203. The mechanism of injury for bursitis is
a. depression of the area.
b. traumatic compression.
c. repeated movement of the area.
d. lack of electrolytes.
e. decrease in reabsorption ability.

204. Nystagmus is a sign of
a. an eye injury.
b. a head injury.
c. a nose injury.
d. anterior compartment syndrome.
e. shoulder dislocation.

205. Retrograde anemia is associated with which type(s) of head injury?
a. First-degree concussion
b. Second and third-degree concussions
c. Jaw injuries
d. Cranial nerve disruption
e. Throat injury

206. In what instance can confidentiality be broken for the purpose of immediate referral?
a. Use of drugs
b. Neurotic behavior
c. Sexual liaisons
d. Suicide possibility
e. Contagious disease

207. When should an athlete be referred for counseling?
a. Anytime there is a neurosis
b. When surgery is needed
c. If an injury recovery will be delayed
d. After the death of a parent
e. If the athlete asks for one

208. An athlete with a head injury presents with difficulty speaking. Which cranial nerve has been affected?
a. V trigeminal
b. VII facial
c. IX glossopharyngeal
d. X vagus
e. XII hypoglossal

209. An athlete has worn his hard contacts for an extended period of time. After removing lenses he is suffering from photophobia and tearing. What do you suspect the athlete is suffering from?

a. Sty
b. Conjunctivitis
c. Corneal abrasion
d. Corneal laceration
e. Detached retina

210. A field hockey player was struck in the eye with a ball. She reports that she sees sparks. You should suspect she suffers from a
a. "blowout" fracture.
b. cataract.
c. concussion.
d. detached retina.
e. corneal laceration.

211. A wrestler is "head butted" just beneath his eye. He immediately retires from the match, holding his eye. Examination reveals inability to move the eye symmetrically, and he reports diplopia. You suspect what injury?
a. Corneal abrasion
b. Corneal laceration
c. Hyphema
d. Sinus fracture
e. "Blowout" fracture

212. A wrestler has received numerous blows to her outer ear. If she continues to avoid use of headgear she will likely suffer
a. hearing loss.
b. concussion.
c. otitis externa.
d. pinna hematoma ("cauliflower ear").
e. otitis media.

213. When evaluating an athlete with a suspected nasal fracture, the evaluation must be extensive enough to eliminate what injury?
a. Skull fracture
b. Epistaxis
c. Fractured teeth
d. Dislocated mandible
e. Neck injury

214. A diet deficient of niacin will result in what problem for the athlete?
a. Anemia
b. Excessive bruising
c. Lack of energy
d. Kidney stones
e. Skin problems

215. An athlete tests positive for a Battle's sign within a few minutes of being injured. You suspect
a. an injury to the forearm.
b. an injury of the anterior humerus.
c. a bruise.
d. dislocated mandible.
e. skull fracture.

216. A mechanism of the head in which the injury occurs opposite the actual site of initial impact is called
a. focal injury.
b. contrecoup injury.
c. direct injury.
d. diffuse injury.
e. stress-strain injury.

217. Which mechanism of injury is most likely to result in death via head injury?
a. Focal
b. Contrecoup
c. Direct
d. Diffuse
e. Stress-strain

218. Skull fractures depend on several factors, including
a. direction of impact, surrounding structures, muscle activity, and perception of athlete.
b. nutrition, age, gender, and time of day.
c. size of area, thickness of bone, material makeup of bone, and amount of impact.
d. amount of hair, area of skull, size of impact, and if it is a game.
e. weather condition, thickness of bone, velocity of object, and fitness of athlete.

219. A soccer goalie dives for a ball and is kicked in the face. She was wearing her mouth guard. She has malocclusion, discoloration under her tongue, and a one-centimeter bleeding separation between two teeth. You suspect a
a. mandibular fracture.
b. maxilia fracture.
c. tooth fracture.
d. temporomandibular dislocation.
e. tooth intrusion.

220. A sign of a maxillary fracture is
a. ecchymosis.
b. diploma.
c. hyphema.
d. tinnitus.
e. temporomandibular joint dysfunction.

221. A seasonal allergy of the upper respiratory tract that causes sneezing, watery eyes, and a runny nose is known as
a. pharyngitis.
b. common cold.
c. hay fever.
d. sinusitis.
e. bronchitis.

222. A bacterial infection of the ear canal found frequently among swimmers is
a. otitis media.
b. otitis externa.
c. "cauliflower ear" (pinna hematoma).
d. impacted cerumen.
e. serous otitis.

223. Plantar's warts (verrucae plantaris) are found
a. on the plantar aspect of the foot.
b. on the dorsal aspect of the foot.
c. on the palmar aspect of the hand.
d. on the dorsal aspect of the hand.
e. on the plantar aspect of the foot and palmar aspect of the hand.

224. A subacromial bursitis, in a pitcher, will be indicated if which signs and symptoms are present?
a. Pain during follow-through phase
b. Pain when sleeping on affected shoulder and during acceleration phase

c. Pain with passive flexion from 90 to 120 degrees
d. Pain with passive extension from 20 to 50 degrees
e. Pain with internal rotation

225. Which nerve is injured if there is winging of the scapula?
a. Axillary
b. Radial
c. Median
d. Long thoracic
e. Ulnar

226. The winging of the scapula can result from which muscle being weak?
a. Deltoid
b. Infraspinatus
c. Trapezium
d. Supraspinatus
e. Serratus anterior

227. A dislocation of the shoulder may damage the glenoid labrum. This is known as a
a. posterior dislocation.
b. Bankart lesion.
c. second-degree tear.
d. positive McMurray test.
e. first-time dislocation.

228. Which manual techniques can be used by the athletic trainer to determine if there is a fracture of the forearm or upper arm?
a. X-ray and tuning fork
b. Observation and inspection
c. History
d. Compression, percussion, distraction, and palpation
e. Muscle testing

■ *Immediate Care*

Directions: Each of the questions or incomplete statements here is followed by five suggested answers or completions. Select the best answer in each case.

229. A rapid thready pulse is an indication of
a. shock.
b. poison.
c. liver disease.
d. anemia.
e. low blood pressure.

230. A slow pulse can be caused by
a. shock.
b. head injury.
c. high blood pressure.
d. fever.
e. cardiac arrest.

231. An athlete who has a reddish skin color is indicating
a. blood loss.
b. heart attack.
c. frost bite.
d. liver disease.
e. high blood pressure.

232. If an athlete is wheezing this is an indication of what abnormality?
a. Shock
b. Head injury
c. Partial airway obstruction
d. Hyperventilation
e. Asthma

233. Normal adult respiratory rate is
a. 6 to 100.
b. 10 to 12.
c. 12 to 20.

d. 60 to 80.
e. 80 to 100.

234. Rapid shallow breathing is an indication of what problem?
a. Lack of oxygen
b. Allergic reaction
c. Chest injury
d. Airway obstruction
e. Too much oxygen

235. An athlete bitten by a bee has self-administered epinephrine via an EpiPen. What vital sign will change as a result?
a. Breathing rate
b. Papillary size
c. Temperature
d. Pulse rate
e. Skin color

236. An athlete with cool and clammy skin is showing signs of
a. cold exposure.
b. shock.
c. pain.
d. heat stroke.
e. fever.

237. Pupils that are lackluster is an indication of
a. head injury.
b. drug overdose.
c. heart attack.
d. shock.
e. stroke.

238. Jaw-thrust maneuver is used when
a. there is a head, neck, or spinal cord injury.
b. there is a jaw injury.
c. there is a partial airway obstruction.
d. there is a throat injury.
e. the athlete is wearing a helmet.

239. Signs that indicate an athlete is in need of Heimlich maneuvers include
a. red faced and unconscious.
b. tearing and coughing.
c. athlete tells you he is choking.
d. look of fear and grabbing his throat.
e. high-pitched whistling.

240. What is the rate of breaths during one-person CPR on an adult?
a. One per second
b. Three per second
c. One per every 5 seconds
d. Two per every 5 seconds
e. Two per every 15 seconds

241. An athlete has an object stuck in the ear canal. What should the athletic trainer recommend?
a. Use a cotton tipped applicator to remove object.
b. Have the athlete shake his head.
c. Have the athlete shake his head, injured ear down.
d. Use an audioscope and view the object before attempting removal.
e. Refer the athlete to physician.

242. When calling 911 for an emergency at work what should the dispatcher be told?

a. What care is being given and how soon emergency care is needed
b. Your name and type of insurance athlete carries
c. How the person was injured
d. How many are injured and nature of injury
e. Your home phone number and what is needed

243. To determine if CPR is effective the athletic trainer will notice
a. constriction of pupils.
b. seizure occurs.
c. heartbeat does not return.
d. athlete remains unresponsive.
e. rigor mortis.

244. When can CPR be interrupted?
a. After 10 minutes of unresponsiveness
b. If there is blood on the lips of the athlete
c. If there are rib fractures that need splinting
d. To check for other injuries
e. To move the athlete onto a stretcher

245. Hypoxia is defined as
a. discoloration of the skin.
b. insufficient supply of oxygen to the tissues.
c. increased supply of oxygen to the tissues.
d. difficulty breathing.
e. difficulty swallowing.

246. How much blood loss must occur in an adult before life is threatened?
a. One quart
b. One pint
c. One liter
d. Two liters
e. Two pints

247. The most effective and quickest way to control external bleeding is
a. direct pressure.
b. elevation.
c. pressure point.
d. tourniquet.
e. pressure bandage.

248. A blood pressure cuff can be used to control life-threatening external bleeding. What is the minimal pressure necessary to control this bleeding?
a. 60 mmHg
b. 90 mmHg
c. 120 mmHg
d. 150 mmHg
e. 180 mmHg

249. A deep bruise on the torso the size of a man's fist is an indication of ____ percent blood loss.
a. 5
b. 10
c. 15
d. 20
e. 25

250. Early signs of shock include
a. weak pulse, vomiting, and anxiety.
b. thirst, nausea, and increased capillary refill.
c. skin color change and decreased respiration.
d. decreased blood pressure, rapid breathing, and weak pulse.
e. fear, increased pulse rate, and restlessness.

251. Which injury would be a priority one life-threatening illness or injury for triage?
   a. Femur fracture without dorsalis pedis pulse
   b. Decapitation
   c. Critical burns without complications
   d. Open fracture of the tibia
   e. A stable drug overdose

252. Which of the following fractures should be cared for first?
   a. Head
   b. Pelvis
   c. Femur
   d. Rib
   e. Spine

253. Ischemia of tissue can occur with a fracture in an extremity. At what point does tissue begin to die?
   a. As soon as fracture occurs
   b. 4 minutes
   c. 6 minutes
   d. 10 minutes
   e. 90 to 120 minutes

254. To treat exercise-induced asthma before activity with inhalant medication (sodium cormoglycate), the medication should be used
   a. 5 minutes before.
   b. 15 minutes before.
   c. 30 minutes before.
   d. 1 hour before.
   e. 4 hours before

255. Expectorants are used to
   a. dry up mucous.
   b. stimulate mucous.
   c. increase the size of the bronchials.
   d. decrease the size of the bronchials.
   e. decrease pain of a sore throat.

256. When removing a contact lens of an unconscious athlete, the athletic trainer should
   a. have the athlete blink.
   b. squeeze the eye from each corner.
   c. take the lens out with fingertips.
   d. trim fingernails before removal.
   e. wear gloves.

257. An athlete has a lacerated tongue and is best treated by
   a. applying ice to the mouth.
   b. applying a dressing and leaning the athlete forward.
   c. packing the mouth full of dressing.
   d. packing the mouth full of dressings and applying a bandage to the mouth.
   e. having the athlete lean head backward.

258. An athlete has received blunt trauma to the throat. Upon examination you feel a crackling sensation under the skin. This is an indication of
   a. cervical spine fracture.
   b. dysphagia.
   c. rib fracture.
   d. subcutaneous emphysema.
   e. tendinitis.

259. The triage system color code for priority four (the lowest priority) is

a. black.
b. red.
c. green.
d. blue.
e. white.

260. An athlete has been cut by a skate. The neck veins have been severed. What is the proper treatment?
a. Apply direct pressure.
b. Elevate the head and apply direct pressure.
c. Elevate the head and apply direct pressure and apply pressure bandage.
d. Apply direct pressure with an occlusive dressing and place athlete on his left side.
e. Apply a tourniquet.

261. The most commonly fractured ribs are the
a. upper four.
b. fifth through tenth.
c. floating.
d. third through sixth.
e. first.

262. When caring for a fractured rib the athletic trainer should
a. place a padded board splint over the rib and bandage the chest.
b. place the injured arm in a sling and swathe.
c. place a sand bag over the site and place the athlete on a spine board injured side up.
d. place ice on the fracture.
e. place an elastic bandage around the chest.

263. What is the initial care for an athlete with a suspected inguinal hernia?
a. Push the hernia back into the abdomen.
b. Apply ice and place the athlete in a position of comfort and refer to a physician.
c. Give the athlete a truss.
d. Apply heat and mild stretching of the abdomen.
e. Full body warm whirlpool and over-the-counter anti-inflammatories.

264. When educating a male athlete regarding side-effects of steroids, include information about
a. increase in muscle bulk size.
b. deepening of the voice.
c. osteoporosis and predisposition for fractures.
d. diabetes.
e. seizure disorder.

265. A femur fracture is best splinted using
a. a backboard.
b. traction splint.
c. vacuum splint.
d. board splint.
e. knee immobilizer.

266. When dealing with an unconscious athlete having a diabetic emergency the immediate care is to
a. lay athlete on his side and place a small amount of sugar under his tongue.
b. give the athlete orange juice.

c. call the athlete's parents for advice.
d. leave the athlete alone as he will recover spontaneously.
e. call a physician for advice.

267. Manual traction or tension being applied to a tibial is done

a. when it is compound.
b. when the splint will be applied immediately thereafter.
c. after ice is applied to numb the area.
d. if fracture is in alignment.
e. when athlete is in shock.

268. An athlete reports acute abdominal pain. She is lying on her side with her knees flexed. What is the best care for this athlete?

a. Treat for shock, lay her supine, straighten her legs, and transport to a local hospital.
b. Treat for shock, lay her supine, keep knees flexed, and transport to a local hospital.
c. Cover athlete with a blanket, monitor vitals, and watch for vomiting.
d. Cover athlete with a blanket, give some food and water, and reassure.
e. Cover athlete with a blanket, give antacid medication, and monitor; if not better refer to physician.

269. If an athlete has a lot of itching, what drug class will likely be prescribed for treatment?

a. Antidotes
b. Irritants
c. Antipruritics
d. Carminatives
e. Emetics

270. An athlete is considered to have high blood pressure when there is a pressure reading

a. below 90.
b. 120/80.
c. 150/90.
d. 60/90.
e. above 160.

271. A softball player slides into home and lime goes into the left eye. What is the first aid care?

a. Neutralize lime with vinegar.
b. Neutralize lime with baking soda.
c. Cover both eyes and transport to the emergency room.
d. Rinse left eye from nose side outward.
e. Rinse left eye from outward toward nose.

272. Which form of heat emergency has the following signs/symptoms: weakness, skin is moist and warm, perspiration is heavy and there are muscle cramps?

a. Heat stroke
b. Heat exhaustion
c. Heat cramps

d. Hyperthermia
e. Hypothermia

273. When should a backboard be used?
a. To immobilize spinal cord injury
b. When it is necessary to elevate the feet
c. When carrying someone down a narrow hall
d. When carrying someone down a curving hall
e. When the person is vomiting

274. A scoop style stretcher
a. should not be used to transport spinal cord–injured patients.
b. should be used in narrow halls.
c. should be used in curving halls.
d. should be used when the person is having a seizure.
e. should be used for victims in shock.

275. An athlete is hit in the eye. The aqueous humor is spilling. What is the immediate care?
a. Patch the eye with a protective shield and transport to hospital.
b. Patch the eye and monitor for 24 to 48 hours.
c. Rinse the eye with saline solution.
d. Place a cup under the eye and transport to hospital.
e. Backboard the athlete.

276. An athlete has a foreign object in his eye. You are unable to locate the object after a thorough examination. The next step is to
a. patch that eye and refer to a physician.
b. patch both and refer to a physician.
c. use copious amounts of water to rinse the eye.
d. have another person look for the object.
e. darken the room lighting and use a penlight to visualize the field.

277. The immediate care for a sty is to
a. patch the eye and refer to a physician.
b. patch both eyes and refer to a physician.
c. aspirin, decongestant, and rest.
d. referral to a physician.
e. moist hot compresses for 48 hours.

278. An athlete has diarrhea. What over-the-counter drug would you recommend?
a. Phenergan
b. Imodium AD
c. Milk of magnesia
d. Tagament
e. Lomotil

279. The immediate treatment for a temporomandibular joint dislocation is to
a. wrap jaw in a bandage and refer to a physician.
b. apply heat and refer to a physician.
c. apply downward and posterior pressure to gain relocation.

d. apply upward and posterior pressure to gain relocation.
e. refer to a physician.

280. Which loose tooth should be placed back in normal position by the athletic trainer?
a. Partially displaced laterally outwardly
b. Intrusion
c. Luxation
d. Fracture
e. Partially displaced laterally, outwardly, or inwardly

281. The immediate care for a fractured tooth with a small exposed area of pulp is
a. place a sterile gauze around the tooth.
b. apply a sterile gauze and have athlete hold milk in his mouth until seen by dentist.
c. wear a mouth guard until seen by a dentist.
d. apply ice and refer to dentist.
e. refer to dentist.

282. When preserving a dislocated tooth, the athletic trainer may
a. scrub dirt off the tooth.
b. wait up to 24 hours before getting athlete to dentist.
c. relocate tooth if it can be done gently.
d. place tooth in his mouth.
e. relocate tooth only if it is in the anterior portion of the mouth.

283. A first-time shoulder dislocation should receive what immediate care from the athletic trainer?
a. Immobilize and refer to a physician.
b. Relocate the shoulder if it can be done gently.
c. Relocate the shoulder after applying ice.
d. Apply heat and refer to a physician.
e. Have the athlete forcefully move into adduction and internal rotation.

284. The athletic trainer should give what type of first aid for an intruded tooth?
a. Push tooth back into socket.
b. Pull tooth back into the socket.
c. Take tooth out and place under tongue for dentist to repair.
d. Place in milk and give to dentist for placement.
e. Refer to dentist, no immediate care is necessary.

285. An athlete has an infected wound with red streaks that travel proximally. The athletic trainer should care for this wound by
a. cleaning with antibacterial soap.
b. applying antibiotic ointment.
c. applying a dressing and recommending aspirin for pain.

d. applying a hot compress 10 minutes an hour.
e. referring to a physician as soon as possible.

286. Splinting of a temporomandibular joint dislocation or a mandibular fracture can be accomplished using a
a. mouth guard.
b. Philadelphia collar.
c. soft collar.
d. padded board and bandage.
e. vacuum splint.

287. The care for a fracture of the clavicle is
a. ice but not splint.
b. ice and splint.
c. place in a shoulder harness.
d. place in a sling with a swathe.
e. heat and placed in a sling with a swathe.

288. The care for an athlete with severe hypothermia who has a heartbeat is to
a. cover with blankets, elevate feet, and call for an ambulance.
b. immerse in warm water and call for an ambulance.
c. give mouth-to-mouth recusitation and call for an ambulance.
d. place near a heater, monitor vital signs, and call for an ambulance.
e. give warmed alcohol to drink, cover with a blanket, and monitor periodically.

289. The athletic trainer should be able to remove a face mask in
a. 30 seconds.
b. 2 minutes.
c. 3 minutes.
d. 4 minutes.
e. 4-6 minutes.

290. The American Psychiatric Association principles on emergency emotional care dictates
a. accepting personal limitations.
b. accepting the death of the athlete.
c. show pity to the injured athlete.
d. disassociation with personal feelings.
e. not personalizing so other athletes can be treated.

291. If the athletic trainer does not have the ability to cut the plastic clips on a football face mask and the athlete is not breathing, it is best to
a. use a straw.
b. use the barrel of a pen.
c. use a pocket mask with a mouthpiece.
d. remove the helmet.
e. blow air into athlete's face.

292. The immediate care for a fractured tooth with a small exposed area of pulp is to
a. place a sterile gauze around the tooth.
b. apply a sterile gauze and have athlete hold milk in his mouth until seen by dentist.

c. wear a mouth guard until seen by a dentist.
d. apply ice and refer to dentist.
e. refer to dentist.

293. When preserving a dislocate tooth, the athletic trainer may
a. scrub dirt off the tooth.
b. wait up to 24 hours before getting athlete to dentist.
c. relocate tooth if it can be done gently.
d. place tooth in his mouth.
e. relocate tooth only if it is in the anterior portion of the mouth.

294. The immediate care for an athlete with a dislocated patella is to
a. extend the knee to relocate the patella.
b. flex the knee to relocate the patella.
c. heat, compress, immobilize, and refer to a physician.
d. ice, compress, immobilize, and refer to a physician.
e. have the athlete walk on it.

295. Acute anterior compartment syndrome is immediately treated by
a. splinting.
b. ice and compression wrap.
c. heat and compression wrap.
d. immediate referral to physician.
e. ice and range of motion exercises.

296. A 20-minute application of cold will
a. increase blood flow.
b. decrease endothelial cell collection.
c. increase vascular spasm.
d. increase blood pressure.
e. increase hemorrhaging.

297. To reduce hypoxia after an acute injury
a. apply cold immediately.
b. apply cold whirlpool immediately.
c. have the athlete continuously move the body part.
d. apply analgesic balm.
e. apply hydrocullator pack.

298. The best opportunity to evaluate an acute injury is within the
a. first few minutes.
b. first hour.
c. first 3 hours.
d. first 12 hours.
e. first 24 hours.

299. To reduce scarring in a wound that requires skin closures, it should be closed within
a. 6 hours.
b. 8 hours.
c. 12 hours.
d. 24 hours.
e. 48 hours.

300. When applying 20 minutes of cold to an injured area, what is the minimum time that the part be rewarmed before cooling a second time?
a. 0 minutes
b. At least 10 minutes
c. At least 10 minutes and cold application no longer

than 10 minutes the second time
d. At least 20 minutes
e. At least 40 minutes

301. To be most effective, a bag of ice is applied
a. over a towel.
b. over an elastic bandage.
c. over a salt solution.
d. directly to the skin.
e. with a large amount of air in the bag.

302. Cold-chemical packs are contraindicated
a. when there is inflammation.
b. after 24 to 72 hours.
c. with an elastic compression bandage.
d. if less than 10 minutes.
e. in a chronic injury.

303. Continuous cryotherapy will cause frostbite when applied longer than
a. 20 minutes.
b. 30 minutes.
c. 40 minutes.
d. 60 minutes.
e. if rewarming is allowed.

304. Medicated ice is used for
a. rapid melting of ice.
b. open abrasion with hemorrhaging.
c. open wounds requiring stitches.
d. preventing ice from transferring viral infection.
e. increasing skin temperature in those with previous history of frostbite.

305. To decrease an athlete's fear after an injury the athletic trainer should tell the athlete
a. the plan to get him back and the duration of injury.
b. "No problem: I've dealt with this before."
c. "Don't worry. I've seen worse."
d. "Even injured, you're better than the back-up."
e. "I understand how you feel. Here's what I can do to help."

306. After an initial assessment, the athletic trainer is unsure if a wrist injury is a fracture or sprain. As immediate care, the athletic trainer should
a. send the athlete for x-ray.
b. wrap the wrist with an elastic bandage.
c. tape the wrist.
d. apply ice and assess in an hour.
e. splint the wrist.

307. Air splints can gain pressure after application if
a. there is a cooler temperature change.
b. there is a warmer temperature change.
c. there is an air leak.
d. there is a valve leak.
e. the zipper comes undone.

308. An athlete has a dislocation with no distal pulse. The immediate care is
a. relocate the dislocation.
b. apply a traction splint.

c. splint and send to emergency room immediately.
d. treat fro shock.
e. elevate the body part and then splint.

309. Treatment for folliculitis is
a. hot compresses.
b. antihistamines.
c. stop shaving.
d. gentle washing and dabbing area.
e. astringents and antibiotics.

310. After an emergency situation, the chart that documents the injury reads "CC sharp pain R BK MD to R O FX." This means
a. cubic centimeter sharp pain, range blocked, medical diagnosis to review family history.
b. cubic centimeter sharp pain of the right back, medical diagnosis to rule out fever.
c. carbon copy of sharp pain, from family history, the right back, need medical diagnosis to rule our fracture.
d. complains of sharp pain in the right back, medical side needed to record frequency.
e. chief complaint sharp pain, right, below knee, medical doctor to rule out fracture.

311. An athletic trainer has been called to the scene of an athlete who is physically violent while under the influence of drugs. The athletic trainer should
a. restrain the athlete.
b. talk calmly and tell the athlete about dangers of abuse.
c. gather many people together to restrain the athlete.
d. move to a safe place and call the police.
e. determine the drug and get an antidote.

312. Direct pressure is best for controlling bleeding because
a. it stops bleeding from a vein.
b. it stops bleeding from an artery.
c. it stops bleeding at that site.
d. it works with gravity to decrease pressure.
e. it stops the blood supply from getting to the site of injury.

313. When applying a splint with an open wound
a. cover the wound with sterile, dry dressing before splinting.
b. cover the wound with sterile, dry dressing after splinting.
c. leave the wound uncovered so it is easily identified.
d. place a note on the splint noting wound.
e. apply pressure to the artery above the site until bleeding stops.

314. When splinting a fracture of the midshaft tibia, immobilize the fracture

a. 2 inches above and below the site.
b. 10 inches above and below the site.
c. hip and foot and the site.
d. foot and hip and the site.
e. ankle and knee and the site.

315. Pillows, air, and vacuum are examples of
a. rigid splints.
b. traction splints.
c. soft splints.
d. spinal splints.
e. aluminum splints.

316. Circulation and neurological status are checked when there is a fracture
a. before splinting.
b. after splinting.
c. before and after splinting.
d. only if there is swelling.
e. only if there is decreased motion.

317. An athlete has a penetrating impaled object. The athletic trainer should care for the injury by
a. removing the object while applying direct pressure.
b. applying direct pressure to the object to stop the bleeding.
c. applying direct pressure to the side of the object to stop the bleeding.
d. applying skin closures upon removal of the object.
e. applying a bandage over the impaled object with excessive pressure.

318. The athletic trainer notices that an athlete has pinpoint pupils, decreased pulse rate, and shallow breathing. Another athlete reports that her friend took some drugs before she started having problems. What drug has been abused?
a. Hallucinogens
b. Depressants
c. Stimulants
d. Narcotics
e. Inhalants

319. An object has impaled the cheek of an athlete. When should the object be removed?
a. Only when it can be done easily
b. Never
c. Only when it can be twisted for easy removal
d. If there is bleeding
e. If the athlete is in pain

320. To ensure that a shock from an automatic defibrillator is delivered to the heart, it is best to
a. make sure the skin is clean and dry.
b. position pads on the center of the chest and right side.
c. position pads on the center of the chest and over the heart.
d. position pads on the center of the chest and over the left shoulder.
e. position pads over the left and right sides just below the armpits.

321. The athletic trainer has administered a third shock to an athlete without heartbeat or respiration. No breathing or heartbeat is present. What is the next course of care administered by the athletic trainer?

a. Another shock
b. Mouth-to-mouth resuscitation
c. Cardiopulmonary resuscitation
d. Precardial thumb
e. Check thrusts

322. Which way should bloody soiled latex gloves be disposed?

a. Disinfect and wash for reuse.
b. Place in bleach solution then place in trash.
c. Place in autoclave.
d. Make sure each glove is inside out and placed in the trash.
e. Place in a biohazard waste bag.

323. A near drowning victim is vomiting up water. What is the immediate care for this victim?

a. Lay victim on his back with hands above his head.
b. Elevate the athlete's legs and hips.
c. Elevate the athlete's head.
d. Roll the victim on his side.
e. Lay the victim face down with hands above his head.

324. An athlete has severe chest pain. Upon evaluation, the athletic trainer notices that a segment of ribs moves in the opposite direction during normal breathing. What is the immediate care of this athlete?

a. Begin mouth-to-mouth resuscitation.
b. Begin cardiopulmonary resuscitation.
c. Apply a thick pad over the area.
d. Place the athlete on his injured side.
e. Elevate the athlete's head.

325. An athletic trainer has been caring for an open pneumothorax. The athlete begins to have additional problems, including signs of tracheal deviation and distended neck veins. What should the athletic trainer do immediately?

a. Call for an ambulance.
b. Check to make sure an occlusive dressing has a valve to allow air release.
c. Apply an occlusive dressing and seal all sides.
d. Place athlete so injured side is up.
e. Place athlete so injured side is down.

326. An athlete has a second-degree burn. What is the care given by the athletic trainer?

a. Apply antibiotic ointment.
b. Run cold water over the area.
c. Clean with antibacterial soap and water.

d. Have the athlete take aspirin for the pain.
e. Refer to a physician as soon as possible.

327. An athlete reportedly has overdosed on uppers. What is the treatment?
a. Monitor athlete until high is done and refer to counseling.
b. Refer to counseling.
c. Call 9-1-1 emergency, monitor vital signs, and treat for shock.
d. Call 9-1-1 emergency and give caffeine.
e. Call 9-1-1 emergency and give alcohol.

328. An athlete has a first time shoulder dislocation. The athletic trainer should care for the dislocation by
a. checking the pulse and nerve function, then placing the arm in a sling and swathing and referring to a physician for care.
b. splinting the clavicle and glenohumeral joint, then placing in a sling and swathing and referring to a physician for care.
c. placing a weight in the athlete's hand, internally rotating the shoulder to relocate it.
d. placing a weight in the athlete's hand, externally rotating the shoulder to relocate it.
e. placing ice on the shoulder and referring to a physician for care.

329. A dislocation spontaneously reduces. The immediate treatment administered includes
a. referral to a physician if dislocation occurs again.
b. splinting, icing, aspirins, and strengthening exercises.
c. application of heat, immobilization, and range-of-motion exercises.
d. checking distal pulses and nerve function, immobilization, and referral to a physician.
e. applying a bag of ice and recommending rest.

330. The primary sign which indicates the hip is dislocated as opposed to fractured is
a. amount of pain.
b. length of leg.
c. internal rotation.
d. inability to walk.
e. inability to move.

331. The most valid way to determine a leg length discrepancy is
a. an X-ray.
b. measuring from umbilicus to medial malleoli.
c. measuring from anterior iliac spine to medial malleoli.
d. making sure medial malleoli are symmetrical.
e. making sure heels are symmetrical.

332. When is a neck collar placed on an athlete who is supine and has a possible cervical spine injury?
a. Right after the head is stabilized by a rescuer's hands
b. Right after rolling the athlete onto the backboard
c. Right after the head is secured to the backboard
d. Right after the check straps are in place
e. As the first step in the process of backboarding

333. A stair chair is used to transport
a. a person down stairs and through narrow hallways.
b. an unconscious athlete.
c. a disoriented athlete.
d. a supine injured athlete.
e. an athlete in cardiogenic shock.

334. The quarterback of the football team just had the face mask of a defender directly impact the anterior aspect of his knee. Observation reveals the patella is proximal and there is a defect of the patellar tendon. The athletic trainer should suspect
a. patellar tendinitis.
b. patellar tendon rupture.
c. Osgood-Schlatter's disease.
d. chondromalacia patella.
e. patella alta.

335. A swimmer hits his head on the bottom of the pool after the start of a race. The athletic trainer suspects a spinal cord injury. The athletic trainer should
a. backboard the athlete while still in the water.
b. backboard the athlete once on deck.
c. place athlete on a short board while still in the water.
d. place athlete on a short board once on deck.
e. place a life jacket on the athlete to keep his head above water.

336. Epistaxis is most often controlled by
a. pressure applied to nostrils.
b. tilting the head backward.
c. tilting the head forward.
d. applying an astringent.
e. cauterizing.

337. To prevent fibrosis a nasal fracture should be set within
a. 2 days.
b. 5 days.
c. 7 days.
d. 10 days.
e. 14 days.

338. The athletic trainer has determined that an athlete has a fracture of the humerus. How should it be splinted?
a. Use an aluminum splint that runs from the shoulder to the elbow.
b. Use a sling and swathe.
c. Use an aluminum splint that runs from the shoulder to the wrist.
d. Use two padded boards that run from the shoulder to the elbow.

e. Straighten the elbow and strap the arm against the body.

339. An athlete has a temperature of 102 degrees F. What is the treatment for this athlete?

a. Give athlete pseudoephedrine tablets and rest.
b. Give athlete acetaminophen tablets and rest.
c. Give athlete acetaminophen tablets and allow participation.
d. Refer to a physician.
e. Apply cold packs to chest and neck.

340. The mechanism of injury for a brachial plexus "burner" is

a. a fall upon an outstretched hand.
b. a fall upon the tip of the shoulder.
c. a lateral blow to the shoulder.
d. downward pressure on the shoulder with the head going away from that shoulder.
e. downward pressure on the shoulder with the head going toward that shoulder.

341. An athlete who is bleeding can have bleeding managed properly in sequence by

a. direct pressure, elevation, then pressure to an artery.
b. direct pressure, elevation, then pressure on a vein.
c. elevation and direct pressure.
d. pressure bandage and elevation.
e. tourniquet.

342. How often is a breath given when performing rescue breathing on an adult?

a. 20 per minute
b. 12 per minute
c. 7 to 10 per minute
d. 5 per minute
e. 3 per minute

343. When treating heat exhaustion allow the athlete to

a. drink salt water.
b. drink ice water.
c. drink cold water.
d. drink cool water.
e. rest in cool place.

344. Which heat disorder requires monitoring of body weight?

a. Heat cramps
b. Heat exhaustion
c. Heat stroke
d. Heat syncope
e. Heat stroke and exhaustion

345. Before giving an athlete an over-the-counter drug, determine his

a. age.
b. height.
c. weight.
d. gender.
e. allergies.

346. When assessing an athlete's pulse in a medical emergency, the primary site of palpation is the

a. jugular vein.
b. radial artery.
c. carotid artery.

d. dorsalis pedis artery.
e. brachial artery.

347. The carotid artery is located
a. on the medial aspect of the upper arm.
b. between the cricoid and the thyroid cartilage.
c. posterior of the sternocleidomastoid.
d. on the lateral aspect of the neck.
e. between the sternocleidomastoid and the larynx.

348. When moving an athlete down a flight of stairs on a stretcher, remember to
a. keep the head end higher.
b. keep the foot end higher.
c. keep the stretcher level.
d. use additional blankets for cushioning.
e. tighten the stretcher straps so the athlete will not shift.

349. An incomplete fracture commonly found in children is known as
a. stress fracture.
b. epiphyseal fracture.
c. greenstick fracture.
d. pathologic fracture.
e. displaced fracture.

350. An athlete in a diabetic coma requires what treatment?
a. Sugar under his tongue
b. An injection of insulin
c. Administration of codeine
d. Administration of histamine-2 blockers
e. Administration of amphetatmines

351. In an initial injury the preferred modality is
a. a cold whirlpool.
b. a cold bath with ice.
c. ice.
d. ultrasound.
e. electrical stimulation.

352. Ice application to an acute injury decreases pain because of
a. decreased physical activity.
b. decreased neurological activity.
c. decreased neurological activity of thermoreceptors.
d. stimulation of endorphins.
e. stimulation of enkephalins.

353. A severely injured athlete has the greatest chance of survival if he receives
a. specialized care within an hour.
b. cardiopulmonary resuscitation.
c. shock care at the scene.
d. medication at the scene.
e. airway protection at the scene.

354. Ice massage is applied until
a. skin is numb.
b. skin is cold.
c. hurting response occurs.
d. 20 minutes passes.
e. pain free.

355. Ice immersion is contraindicated for acute injury because
a. it is too cold.
b. it covers more area than the injury.

c. temperature is inconsistent.
d. body part is in a gravity-dependent position.
e. the ice causes pressure injury.

356. The most effective modality used to decrease edema is
a. ice.
b. ice and elastic bandage.
c. ice and elastic bandage and elevation.
d. intermittent compression.
e. cold and compression unit.

■ *Treatment, Rehabilitation, and Reconditioning*

Directions: Each of the questions or incomplete statements here is followed by five suggested answers or completions. Select the best answer in each case.

357. An athlete psychologically is at risk for injury when there is
a. a previous injury.
b. a lack of motivation.
c. he is physically out of shape.
d. pressure to perform.
e. fewer practice minutes.

358. Which modality has the deepest penetration?
a. Lasers
b. Shortwave diathermy
c. Hot whirlpool
d. Paraffin bath
e. Cold whirlpool

359. A closed-kinetic-chain isometric wrist extension exercise is
a. wrist curls.
b. free weight wrist extensions.
c. dumbbell incline bench press.
d. hammer curls.
e. push-ups.

360. Cosine law states that
a. for every action there is an equal and opposite reaction.
b. no changes occur in tissue because the amount of energy is not being absorbed.
c. more energy will be absorbed the closer the energy source is to a right angle.
d. energy not absorbed superficially will penetrate deeper.
e. longer wavelength radiation will absorb deeper.

361. Which electrical stimulating current helps soft tissue and bone heal by using subsensory microcurrents?
a. Ultrasound
b. Direct current
c. Alternating current
d. TENS
e. MENS

362. Which modality is used for muscle re-education?
a. Low-voltage electrical stimulation
b. High-voltage electrical stimulation

c. Biofeedback
d. TENS
e. MENS

363. The cellular removal of damaged cells, resulting from injury, is done by
a. application of cold.
b. application of heat.
c. red blood cells.
d. phagocytes.
e. plasma.

364. Effusion of blood at the site of an acute injury occurs for
a. 20 minutes.
b. 6 hours.
c. 24 to 36 hours.
d. 2 weeks.
e. 6 weeks.

365. Which chemical mediators are responsible for increased cell permeability after injury?
a. Histamine and leucotaxin
b. Necrosin and histamine
c. Fibrinogen and thrombin
d. Prothrombin and fibrinogen
e. Fibrinogen and thromboplastin

366. The inflammatory response lasts
a. 20 minutes.
b. 24 to 48 hours.
c. 48 to 96 hours.
d. 2 weeks.
e. 6 weeks.

367. In clot formation, what causes prothrombin to change into thrombin?
a. Fibrinogen
b. Thromboplastin
c. Histamine
d. Platelets
e. Leukocytes

368. Chronic inflammation occurs because of
a. repeated injury to the tissue.
b. failure of phagocytes to clear injured tissue.
c. the area is highly vascularized.
d. muscular contractions around the area.
e. lack of clot formation at the injury site.

369. Capillary buds grow in a wound because of
a. lack of blood.
b. lack of nutrients.
c. lack of oxygen.
d. excess fat.
e. excess blood pressure.

370. Analgesics work by
a. decreasing swelling.
b. vasodialation of vessels and stopping prostaglandin production.
c. transmitting sensory information to the brain.
d. blocking motor transmission.
e. blocking sensory transmission.

371. Keloids occur because of
a. a lack of vitamin E.
b. infection.
c. collagen build-up exceeds collagen break-down.
d. improper nutrition.
e. major tissue injury.

372. Lack of vitamin K affects wound healing because it

a. decreases chemical mediators.
b. decreases amino acids.
c. decreases clotting ability.
d. decreases collagen.
e. thins the blood.

373. An example of isotonic open-kinetic-chain strengthening for the iliopsoas is
a. hip extension, straight leg raises with weights.
b. hip abduction, straight leg raises with weights.
c. hip adduction, straight leg raises with weights.
d. hip flexion, straight leg raises with weights.
e. knee extensions with weights.

374. Ultrasound used with an acute injury will
a. increase swelling.
b. decrease pain.
c. decrease spasm.
d. decrease swelling.
e. allow sodium and calcium ions to pass into cells.

375. To prevent a low back strain, an athlete should be taught to
a. keep shoulders over feet, avoiding rotation.
b. keep his head down.
c. make sure he inherits good genes.
d. wear rib protection.
e. increase lordosis posture.

376. Transverse friction massage is recommended for
a. release of endorphins.
b. increased circulation.
c. decreasing pain.
d. decreasing edema.
e. increasing adhesions.

377. An athlete is in need of isometric ankle inversion exercise. Where should the athletic trainer give resistance?
a. On the medial malleolus
b. On the medial portion of the foot
c. On the lateral malleolus
d. On the lateral portion of the foot
e. On the plantar surface of the foot

378. High-voltage electrical stimulation is indicated
a. for fracture healing.
b. to decrease blood flow.
c. to reduce inflammation.
d. to increase tissue temperature.
e. to increase analgesia.

379. When progressing through rehabilitation muscular strength must be obtained before
a. agility and joint integrity.
b. speed and pain-free joints.
c. cardiovascular endurance and power.
d. muscular endurance and flexibility.
e. sport-specific skills and pain-free muscles.

380. Thermotherapy is contraindicated if there is
a. a metal implant.
b. poor neurological response.
c. poor circulation.
d. skin sensitivities.
e. an open wound.

381. **Wound healing is best facilitated by which modalities?**
   a. TENS, cold packs, and infrared lamps.
   b. High-voltage electrical stimulation, diathermy and thermo-therapy.
   c. Ultrasound, ultraviolet light, and interferential electrical stimu-lation.
   d. MENS, low-power laser, and low-voltage electrical stimulation.
   e. Intermittent compression, hydrocullator packs, and ultrasound.

382. **Decreased edema is best accomplished using**
   a. ultrasound.
   b. high-voltage electrical stimulation.
   c. intermittent compression.
   d. cryotherapy.
   e. thermotherapy.

383. **A contraindication of intermittent compression is**
   a. infection.
   b. acute injury.
   c. circulatory problems.
   d. sensitivity.
   e. loss of sensation.

384. **Which of the following tissues is least sensitive to painful stimuli?**
   a. Articular cartilage
   b. Periosteum
   c. Tendons
   d. Bone
   e. Muscle

385. **Which tissue is most sensitive to painful stimuli?**
   a. Ligament
   b. Bone
   c. Tendon
   d. Synovium
   e. Periosteum

386. **Proprioceptors respond to**
   a. pain.
   b. pressure.
   c. temperature.
   d. light.
   e. tension.

387. **Corpuscles of Ruffini are located in**
   a. blood vessels.
   b. hair follicles.
   c. skin.
   d. muscle.
   e. heart.

388. **Nociceptors function to sense**
   a. temperature.
   b. pain.
   c. pressure.
   d. tension.
   e. light.

389. **Meissner's corpuscles respond to**
   a. temperature.
   b. tension.
   c. light touch.
   d. deep touch.
   e. hair movement.

390. **Which nerve fibers transmit sensory impulses to the brain?**
   a. Afferent
   b. Mechanoreceptors
   c. Thermoreceptors
   d. Dermatomes
   e. Efferent

391. **Resistance tubing placed on the forefoot with eversion motion will strengthen which muscles?**

a. Peroneus longus, brevis, and tertius
b. Extensor digitorum longus and plantaris
c. Posterior tibialis and flexor hallicus longus
d. Flexor digitorum longus and soleus
e. Gastrocnemius and anterior tibialis

392. Athletes who have chronic pain may
a. learn to tolerate the pain and disability.
b. have an overabundance of serotonin release.
c. become depressed, lose sleep, and have decreased appetite.
d. have damaged neuropathways.
e. have reduced ability to produce neurotransmitters.

393. Spoon-shaped nails result from
a. poor nutrition.
b. compression injury.
c. fungus infection.
d. bacterial infection.
e. paronychia.

394. Nail clubbing results from
a. enlargement of the soft tissue.
b. severe illness.
c. iron deficiency.
d. fungus infection.
e. warts.

395. Scoliosis is due to right musculature on the
a. same side of the curve.
b. opposite side of the curve.
c. anterior side of the curve.
d. anterior and same as the curve.
e. anterior and opposite side of the curve.

396. Body parts commonly affected by frostbite are
a. cheeks, fingertips, and toes.
b. cheeks, thighs, fingertips, and toes.
c. cheeks, forehead, nose, and fingertips.
d. fingertips, toes, and earlobes.
e. fingertips, dorsal of hands, and nose.

397. Trigger finger is a result of
a. avulsion of the extensor tendon.
b. flexor tendon nodule.
c. a tear in the annular sheath.
d. repetitive flexion.
e. congenital abnormality.

398. An apparent leg-length discrepancy is determined by measuring from
a. anterior superior iliac spine to medial femoral condyle.
b. medial femoral condyle to lateral malleolus.
c. anterior superior iliac spine to medial malleolus.
d. umbilicus to medial malleolus.
e. medial tibial plateau to lateral malleolus.

399. In the late stages of rehabilitation it is psychologically important that
a. the athlete is able to endure more pain.

b. the athlete keeps his sense of humor.
c. goals are set to prevent an injury.
d. range of motion is achieved.
e. the athlete achieves goals for return to play.

400. Signs of suicide include
a. depression, having a plan, and change in behavior.
b. not eating, weight loss, and excessive dieting.
c. obsessive or compulsive behavior.
d. high stress and anxiety.
e. family history of suicide and a positive outlook.

401. When documenting the mental health status of an athlete the athletic trainer should state
a. ability to remember recent events.
b. spatial awareness.
c. physical abilities in a game situation.
d. previous family mental illness.
e. amoral thoughts.

402. Which eating disorder is characterized by amenorrhea?
a. Anorexia nervosa
b. Bulimia nervosa
c. Obesity
d. Anorexia nervosa and bulimia nervosa
e. Bulimia nervosa and obesity

403. When manual resistance is used for finger PIP flexion exercises, which areas are stabilized?
a. Metacarpal phalangeal joint and distal interphalangeal joints.
b. Metacarpal phalangeal joint and proximal interphalangeal joints.
c. Metacarpal phalangeal joint and wrist.
d. Metacarpal phalangeal joint and all other fingers.
e. Distal interphalangeal joint and wrist.

404. When manual resistance is used for thumb adduction, what area is resisted?
a. Wrist and carpometacarpal joint
b. Metacarpal phalangeal joint and metacarpal
c. Distal and proximal interphalangeal joints
d. Wrist and proximal interphalangeal joints
e. Wrist and distal interphalangeal joints

405. Muscle pump contractions can be successful if the current is
a. surging for 5 to 10 seconds.
b. bursting for 5 to 10 seconds.
c. pulsed direct current for 10 to 20 seconds.
d. continuous for 10 to 20 seconds.
e. alternating for 10 to 20 seconds.

406. Reducing muscle atrophy while using electrically stimulated contractions is accomplished using
a. surging current.
b. bursting current.

c. pulsed current.
d. continuous current.
e. ramped current.

407. When using electrical stimulation to create muscular strength, the current is
a. surging current with gradual ramp.
b. bursting current.
c. pulsed current.
d. continuous current.
e. sporadic current.

408. Controlled exercise is important for wound healing because
a. it decreases pain.
b. it decreases swelling.
c. it increases oxygen.
d. it increases agility.
e. it increases pumping action.

409. Functional tests to determine return to competition must evaluate
a. speed, level of skill, agility, and strength.
b. maximal contraction, mental readiness, level of competition, and power.
c. power, strength, ability to use body part, and neuromuscular control.
d. joint laxity, symmetry, proprioception, and strength.
e. coordination, aerobic and anaerobic capacity, and balance.

410. The physiological response to cold therapy is
a. chills.
b. shivering.
c. decrease body temperature.
d. erythema.
e. gray skin color.

411. To increase the workload of wrist flexion being done isometrically do the exercise
a. without weights.
b. while pronated.
c. while supinated.
d. while gripping putty.
e. with gravity.

412. During rehabilitation, an athlete is apprehensive about the injury and return to competition. The athletic trainer can help the athlete by
a. telling him everything will be normal, even if it will not.
b. giving the athlete additional rehabilitation.
c. lowering the rehabilitation goals.
d. allowing the athlete to share feelings and concerns.
e. reassuring the athlete you have dealt with this injury before.

413. Distal humeral traction is used to
a. decrease pain.
b. decrease swelling.
c. increase circulation.
d. increase circumduction.
e. increase external rotation.

414. In a warm whirlpool treatment where there is direct flow upon the body part, the body part should be

a. one to two inches from flow.
b. two to four inches from flow.
c. four to six inches from flow.
d. six to eight inches from flow.
e. eight to ten inches from flow.

415. When using a weight machine for knee extension it is critical to
a. hold his breath on extension.
b. hold his breath on flexion.
c. lift quickly and lower quickly.
d. lift slowly and lower quickly.
e. align the medial of the knee with the cam.

416. The physiological response to thermotherapy includes
a. muscle elongation.
b. pain decrease.
c. tissue temperature increase.
d. numbness.
e. neurological decrease.

417. When should an athlete be referred for counseling?
a. When athlete has good medical coverage
b. When athletic trainer does not have time to talk with athlete
c. When athletic trainer does not have a relationship with the athlete
d. When problem is outside the athletic trainer's scope of practice
e. When problem is morally irritating to the athletic trainer

418. Treatment for folliculitis is
a. hot compresses.
b. antihistamines.
c. stop shaving.
d. gentle washing and dabbing area.
e. astringents and antibiotics.

419. Paraffin in paraffin baths should be replaced
a. biweekly.
b. every week.
c. every 6 months.
d. every 12 months.
e. when half of the paraffin is decreased.

420. The athlete who has been exposed to meningitis is treated by
a. washing hands.
b. immunization.
c. referring to a physician.
d. not doing anything.
e. isolating him.

421. An athlete with pharyngitis/tonsillitis caused by a bacterial infection can return to athletic activity after antibiotics in
a. 2 weeks.
b. 10 days.
c. 1 week.
d. 5 days.
e. 1 to 3 days.

422. The weak muscle involved in chondromalacia is the
a. quadriceps.
b. hamstrings.
c. vastus lateralis.
d. vastus medialis.
e. rectus femoris.

423. Ultrasound can be done
a. no more than 14 times.
b. as often as desired.
c. twice a day for a week.

d. on lower extremities as often as desired, on upper extremities four times.
e. on upper extremities as often as desired, on lower extremities four times.

424. Which of the following is an upper extremity closed kinetic chain exercise?
a. Push-ups
b. Codman's
c. Wall climbs
d. Flies
e. Shoulder shrugs

425. The middle deltoid and supraspinatus can be strengthened by performing isometrics in what range of motion?
a. Internal rotation
b. External rotation
c. Abduction to 90 degrees
d. Adduction and internal rotation
e. Shoulder shrugs

426. Carioca is an example of
a. strength.
b. agility.
c. flexibility.
d. aerobic fitness.
e. anaerobic fitness.

427. Ultrasound is best for which type of tissue?
a. Skin
b. Articular cartilage
c. Vascular
d. Periosteum
e. Fat

428. Plyometric training in the off-season should be done
a. two days per week at maximum capacity, three days per week at half capacity.
b. three days per week at maximum capacity, two days per week at half capacity.
c. three days per week at maximum capacity.
d. five days per week at maximum capacity.
e. seven days per week at maximum capacity.

429. Phonophoresis occurring using immersion is accomplished by applying the medicine
a. to the ultrasonic head.
b. to the body part.
c. to the ultrasonic head and body part.
d. in the water.
e. in the water on the body part and ultrasonic head.

430. Care of chondromalacia patella in an asymptomatic athlete is
a. not necessary.
b. exercise such as squats beyond 90 degrees of flexion.
c. a knee sleeve with a lateral buttress.
d. a knee sleeve with a medial buttress.
e. a knee sleeve with a superior buttress.

431. A massage begins and ends with which stroke?
a. Effleurage
b. Petrissage
c. Friction
d. Tapotement
e. Vibration

432. Petrissage is used to
a. stimulate nerve firing.
b. help the athlete get used to the therapist's touch.
c. break up adhesions.
d. create relaxation.
e. soothe tension.

433. Typical exercise progression is
a. isometrics, isokinetics, isotonics, and functional skills.
b. isokinetics, isotonics, isometrics, and functional skills.
c. isometrics, isotonics, isokinetics, and functional skills.
d. isometrics, isotonics, functional skills, and isokinetics.
e. functional skills, isometrics, isotonics, and isokinetics.

434. Inversion positional traction is contraindicated for
a. scoliosis.
b. disk herniation.
c. high blood pressure.
d. pancreatitis.
e. sickle-cell anemia.

435. Which spinal position allows for the biggest intervertebral foramen opening before traction occurs?
a. Neutral
b. Flexion
c. Extension
d. Lateral flexion
e. Rotation

436. Ringworm is treated with
a. antifungal medication.
b. antibiotics.
c. cleaning area and keeping it moist.
d. anti-yeast medication.
e. aspirin and corticosteroids.

437. Cervical traction is best accomplished in a
a. sitting, bent-kneed position.
b. side lying position.
c. inverted position.
d. supine position.
e. prone position.

438. Manual traction will be enhanced with the addition of
a. electrical stimulation.
b. laser.
c. ice massage.
d. intermittent compression.
e. heating modalities.

439. How long should documentation of mental health records be kept before being destroyed?
a. As soon as athlete leaves program
b. Until athlete is 21 years of age
c. 15 years
d. 30 years
e. The life of the individual

440. Edema caused by injury can cause long-term problems, such as
a. articular degeneration.
b. tendinitis.
c. bursitis.
d. joint contractures.
e. increased blood flow.

441. To aid an athlete psychologically during rehabilitation the athletic trainer should

a. be aggressive, take the athlete off crutches earlier than normal.
b. set up long, short, and daily goals to show progress.
c. talk calmly with the athlete periodically.
d. push the athlete using the "no pain, no gain" theory.
e. push strength early in the plan.

442. Inflation pressure for intermittent compression is
a. 20 mmHg.
b. 30 mmHg.
c. pressure between patient's diastolic and systolic.
d. 120 mmHg.
e. 140 mmHg.

443. Iontophoresis is used to treat
a. pain.
b. atrophy.
c. infection.
d. poor nerve supply.
e. edema.

444. The ion used to treat inflammation in iontophoresis is
a. hydrocortisone.
b. tap water.
c. mineral oil.
d. magnesium.
e. lidocaine.

445. The average duration of iontophoresis is
a. 3 to 5 minutes.
b. 20 minutes on, 20 minutes off and 20 minutes on again.
c. 15 minutes.
d. 20 minutes.
e. 1 hour.

446. Regeneration of tissue in humans
a. is not possible.
b. is possible only in wounds.
c. is possible for tissues that carry only negative currents.
d. is possible for muscle, nerve, bone, skin, and connective tissue.
e. is possible for tissues that carry only positive currents.

447. When using bioelectric current to regenerate cellular growth areas of a wound, remember
a. to keep the wound wet.
b. to let the wound dry out.
c. to have the wound stitched beforehand.
d. to do the wound bilaterally.
e. to keep the current focused on the epidermis, no deeper.

448. Vitamins A and E are important for injury healing, specifically in the area of
a. clothing.
b. phagocytosis.
c. increased blood supply.
d. scarring.
e. collagen synthesis.

449. A wound that will heal the fastest is one that
a. has an infection.
b. is high in humidity.
c. is high in collagen production and decreased collagen breakdown.

d. has poor phagocytosis.
e. has large amount of swelling.

450. The initial ill effects of injury edema include
a. increased cellular death.
b. increased oxygen supply.
c. increased nutrient supply.
d. decreased healing time.
e. decreased intercellular fluid.

451. Pitting edema is the result of
a. an injury to the axilla.
b. an injury to the stomach.
c. an injury to the nail bed.
d. increased extracellular fluid trapped at the site of an injury.
e. increased blood flow away from the site of an injury.

452. Before testing an athlete's level of physical fitness, the testing environment should
a. replicate game conditions.
b. replicate game noise level.
c. be controlled with procedures explained.
d. be about 80 degrees Fahrenheit.
e. be well ventilated and semi-private.

453. Instruction for an athlete before fitness testing should include
a. type of clothing to wear.
b. a copy of the previous test scores.
c. fitness levels of other athletes.
d. risk of exercise.
e. weight loss expected.

454. What equipment requires speed calibration before use?
a. A scale
b. Skin fold calipers
c. Treadmill
d. Thermometer
e. Weighted ball

455. A contraindication of laser use is/are
a. benign tumors.
b. bursitis.
c. pregnancy.
d. facial use.
e. open wounds.

456. The proper hand placement for an athlete performing knee flexion and extension on an isokinetic machine is
a. under the buttocks.
b. grasping the table.
c. on the thighs.
d. across the chest.
e. on the hips.

457. Salicylates used during phonophoresis produce
a. increased analgesia and decreased inflammation.
b. decreased pain.
c. increased blood flow.
d. increased cellular regeneration.
e. increased tissue healing.

458. When performing resistive exercises maximum effort is contra-indicated for what type of injury?
a. Late stage postsurgical ligament repair of the anterior cruciate ligament
b. Late stage femur fracture repair

c. Early stage postsurgical ligament repair of the anterior cruciate ligament
d. Circulatory
e. Neurological

459. Improper rehabilitation will lead to
a. improved functional skills.
b. increased pain.
c. decreased atrophy.
d. weak tissue.
e. improved stability.

460. Resistive exercises are indicated when
a. increased body temperature is desired.
b. decreased pain is necessary.
c. increased endurance is desired.
d. isokinetics do not produce the desired effects.
e. isotonics do not produce the desired effects.

461. Exercise progression occurs in what order?
a. Multiple-angle isometrics, short arc isotonics, and concentric isokinetics
b. Multiple angle isometrics, full range isotonics, and short arc isotonics
c. Full range isokinetics, full range isotonics and isometrics
d. Short arc concentric isokinetics, isometrics, and isokinetics
e. Ice, massage, and exercise

462. Serious knee injuries should avoid being immobilized longer than
a. 24 hours.
b. 48 hours.
c. 3 weeks.
d. 4 weeks.
e. 6 weeks.

463. When documenting a skill deficiency it is best written
a. in complete sentences.
b. in pencil or red ink.
c. by a grouping, i.e. flexibility, strength.
d. longhand.
e. printed by computer.

464. Subjective information in a SOAP note would consist of
a. range of motion, strength, and endurance.
b. aerobic and anaerobic fitness and nutrition.
c. pain, functional capacity, and ability to perform daily skills.
d. history of injury, other medical problems, and current medications.
e. coordination, agility, and family history.

465. Lateral isometric neck flexion is done with resistance applied to the
a. lateral side of flexion.
b. lateral side away from flexion.
c. on the forehead.
d. on the occiput.
e. on the temple.

466. In a mild knee injury, which muscle is most likely to suffer the most atrophy?
a. Vastus medialis
b. Rectus femoris
c. Vastus intermedius
d. Vastus lateralis
e. Sartorius

467. When the knee is immobilized the quadriceps atrophy and the
   a. joint degenerates and the hamstrings atrophy.
   b. patellar articular cartilage softens and the ligaments tighten.
   c. patellar tendon contracts and the ligaments atrophy.
   d. knee becomes painful and the meniscus becomes inflexible.
   e. hamstrings contract and the hip flexor weakens.

468. The quadriceps muscles are at the greatest tension capacity when performing eccentrics at what degree?
   a. 0 degrees
   b. 0 to 30 degrees
   c. 0 to 40 degrees
   d. 30 to 40 degrees
   e. 90 degrees

469. A factor that will affect strength values is
   a. gender.
   b. circulation.
   c. body weight.
   d. ethnicity.
   e. height.

470. An advantage of isotonics over isokinetics is
   a. safer at high speeds.
   b. fiber types change.
   c. variable resistances are accommodated.
   d. accessibility.
   e. synovial joint lubrication.

471. When performing open chained exercises it is likely that there will be
   a. multiple-joint strength carryover.
   b. improved proprioception.
   c. dual joint patterns.
   d. concentric exercises in primary activities.
   e. stabilization occurs in other joints.

472. If an athlete has limited knee flexion and is placed on an exercise bike there will be compensation in the
   a. ankle and hip.
   b. hip and trunk.
   c. hip and pelvis.
   d. ankle and pelvis.
   e. ankle and knee.

473. In the course of rehabilitation a change in plan is necessary when the patient has problems with
   a. an additional injury in another joint.
   b. decreased sensation of the body part and increased strength.
   c. swelling, stiffness, and pain.
   d. dehydration, fatigue, and pain.
   e. increased body temperature, malaise, and headaches.

474. The most economical way to control pain is
   a. TENS.
   b. MENS.
   c. cryotherapy.
   d. high-voltage stimulation.
   e. diathermy.

475. Contractures are a concern if full range of motion does not occur postsurgical knee reconstruction as early as

a. 48 hours.
b. 72 hours.
c. 1 week.
d. 2 to 3 weeks.
e. 3 to 4 weeks.

476. What muscle needs to be activated early in the process of knee rehabilitation to properly align the patella?
a. vastus medialis obliques.
b. vastus intermedius.
c. vastus lateralis.
d. rectus femoris.
e. sartorius.

477. The primary exercise for a knee which is in a knee immobilizer following an acute injury is
a. quadriceps muscle sets.
b. straight leg raises.
c. heel slides.
d. co-contraction of the quadriceps and hamstrings.
e. toe raises.

478. The subacute phase of rehabilitation progression is
a. proprioceptive neuromuscular facilitation.
b. straight leg raises.
c. graduated strengthening exercises.
d. isokinetic muscle exercises.
e. terminal extensions.

479. Overuse injuries occur as a result of what mechanisms of injury?
a. Torsion, direct impact, or friction
b. Repetitive impact, congenital, or muscular imbalances
c. Pronation, supination, or excessive shoe wear
d. Tension, compression, or shearing
e. Increased mileage, angled roads, and excessive weight

480. Cellular atrophy is caused by
a. repetitive stress.
b. fatigue.
c. exercise.
d. chronic inflammation.
e. pain.

481. Which of the following is a functional exercise?
a. Calf raises
b. Lunges
c. Stationary bike
d. Balance board
e. Climbing machine

482. The primary muscle group that should be strengthened for a posterior cruciate ligament injury is
a. hamstrings.
b. quadriceps.
c. adductors.
d. abductors.
e. plantar flexors.

483. The T-drill shuffle test helps determine an athlete's
a. speed.
b. strength.
c. power.
d. agility.
e. endurance.

484. Plyometric training will
a. decrease pain of an acute injury.
b. improve power.
c. improve flexibility.
d. decrease mechanoreceptors.
e. increase agility.

485. Which lower body plyometric training is considered high intensity?
a. Standing jumps
b. Depth jumping
c. In-place jumps
d. Repetitive jumps
e. Sport-specific high-stress drills

486. For an athlete to progress through a figure eight drill, he or she
a. starts with high speed and progresses to low speed.
b. starts with three quarter speed then to slow speed.
c. starts with small figure eight and progresses to bigger ones.
d. starts with shorter distance and progresses to longer.
e. starts with longer distance and progresses to shorter.

487. During functional testing for rehabilitation of a knee the crossover cutting drill is performed by
a. planting a foot and pushing opposite that leg.
b. planting a foot and pushing toward that leg.
c. continuously putting one foot in front of the other.
d. repetitively putting one foot in front then one in back.
e. going at full speed the first time.

488. What should an athlete's heart rate be when using an upper body cycle for the first time for and aerobic workout?
a. 120 beats per minute.
b. 20 percent of maximal heart rate.
c. 40 percent of maximal heart rate.
d. 65 percent of maximal heart rate.
e. 80 percent of maximal heart rate.

■ *Organization and Administration*

Directions: Each of the questions or incomplete statements here is followed by five suggested answers or completions. Select the best answer in each case.

489. Documentation protects whose legal rights?
a. The athlete's
b. The athletic trainer's
c. The athlete and athletic trainer's
d. The athlete's parents
e. The clinic or athletic department

490. Which agency requires documentation of athletic injuries among professional sports athletes in the event of a worker's compensation claim?
a. Occupational Safety and Health Administration (OSHA)
b. Fair Labor Standards
c. National Athletic Trainers' Association Board of Certification (NATABOC)

d. National Football League (NFL)
e. Commission on Accreditation of Rehabilitation Facilities (CARF)

491. When requesting bids for quotation, how many companies should bid?
a. One
b. Two
c. Three
d. Only those who have good reputations
e. Only those who are local

492. Documentation for athletic trainers who work in hospitals is governed by the
a. National Athletic Trainers' Association Board of Certification (NATABOC).
b. Occupational Safety and Health Administration (OSHA).
c. Fair Labor Standards.
d. Joint Commission of Accreditation of Healthcare Organizations.
e. National Association of Hospitals.

493. The principles that guide the activities of an athletic trainer are known as
a. entry-level certification.
b. role delineation.
c. standards of practice.
d. Good Samaritan law.
e. documentation.

494. A drug administration log should include what information?
a. Drug name, date of dispensing, patient name, quantity, name of physician, and intended use
b. Drug name, date of dispensing, patient name, quantity given, complaint, lot number, current medications being taken, drug allergies, date of drug expiration, how drug is administered, and time of administration
c. Date of dispensing, patient name, quantity given, instruction for use, lot number, date of expiration, method administered, and name of physician
d. Patient name, quantity, instruction for use, drug name, date of dispensing, patient name, quantity, half-life of drug, contraindications, warning, drug response, and instructions for use
e. Patient name, quantity, time of day, observers, method administered, copy of prescription, name of drug, and side-effects seen

495. Which information should be a part of an athlete's medical record?
a. Transcripts
b. Quotes
c. Newspaper clippings
d. Academic awards
e. Family records

496. When writing a notation into medical record it must be done
a. double spaced.
b. in chronological order.
c. in red ink.
d. in pencil.
e. when you can.

497. Document the patient's
a. ethnicity.
b. age.
c. sex.
d. complaints.
e. religion.

498. If an error is made in documentation, the correction is made by
a. using correction fluid.
b. erasure.
c. throwing out the recording and starting over.
d. drawing a line through incorrect note(s) and writing correct note(s) next to it.
e. blackening error out with black marker and writing correct note(s) next to it.

499. When leasing equipment, an advantage is
a. overall cost.
b. ownership.
c. decreased obsolescence.
d. lower interest rate.
e. higher interest rate.

500. When a centralized location is not possible for record keeping, facilities
a. use electronic record keeping.
b. allow athletic trainers to keep records with them.
c. allow athlete to keep records with them.
d. use typewriters.
e. use scanners.

501. An advantage of a centralized computer with decentralized settings is
a. that entries are done quickly.
b. that records can be accessed by unauthorized personnel.
c. decreased interaction with patient, but increased output.
d. it is less expensive to update.
e. they rarely are outdated.

502. A patient's medical record should contain
a. treatment records and performance evaluations.
b. physician referrals and insurance pay outs.
c. X-ray reports and freedom of information requests.
d. permission to treat forms and litigation.
e. injury evaluations and physicals.

503. The first record in the medical file of an athlete is typically
a. physical examination.
b. surgical report.
c. authorization to treat.
d. injury evaluation.
e. release of medical information.

504. When planning for a new training room, the square footage is determined by

a. patients divided by tables, multiplied by 100 square feet.
b. patients plus tables, divided by 100 square feet.
c. modality use, plus evaluations, plus taping, multiplied by 100 square feet.
d. modality use, plus taping, multiplied by 100 square feet.
e. patients.

505. Documentation done in which there is data on the injury, the athletic trainer's response, and the athlete's response to care is known as
a. focus charting.
b. computerized documentation.
c. narrative charting.
d. charting by exception.
e. problem-oriented medical records.

506. Hydroptherapy rooms should be equipped with their own
a. air conditioner.
b. furnace.
c. thermostat.
d. drinking fountain.
e. exhaust fan.

507. To free up time when documenting injuries via computer, the athletic trainer can
a. save up records for a one-time entry.
b. hire nonprofessionals.
c. go to narrative charting.
d. just do not document.
e. focus chart and problem-oriented medical record.

508. The traditional method used by athletic trainers to document an injury is
a. focus charting.
b. computerized documentation.
c. narrative charting.
d. charting by exception.
e. problem-oriented medical recording.

509. Dictation is generally used as a part of which type of medical documentation?
a. Focus charting
b. SOAP notes
c. Narrative charting
d. Charting by exception
e. Problem-oriented medical recording

510. Proof that an athlete was seen by a physician is provided by
a. release of medical information.
b. medical referral form.
c. permission to treat form.
d. emergency information form.
e. insurance information form.

511. A medical referral form must allow the physician to
a. release medical information.
b. permission to treat.
c. emergency information.
d. insurance information.
e. age of patient.

512. Emergency information records on athletes who are traveling are to be

a. in a computer database.
b. in each athlete's medical records.
c. with each athlete's parents.
d. at the local hospital.
e. with the team's athletic trainer.

513. Exculpatory clauses should be evaluated by
a. an attorney and insurance carrier.
b. a risk manager.
c. a financial manager.
d. an athletic director.
e. an athletic trainer.

514. Disclosure of medical records to a third party is prevented by
a. standards of practices.
b. ethics of the NATA.
c. Family Educational Rights and Privacy Act.
d. OSHA.
e. NATABOC.

515. When can an athletic trainer release medical information without a signed release?
a. An impending suicide is suspected.
b. A college recruiter is in town.
c. A professional scout is in town.
d. An eating disorder is suspected.
e. A parent is calling.

516. What record is not protected by the Family Educational Rights and Privacy Acts?
a. Physician's referral
b. Treatment log
c. X-rays
d. Insurance information
e. Physical

517. Which of the following is considered a medical record?
a. Equipment purchases
b. Financial insurance claims
c. Patient invoices regarding insurance companies
d. Insurance members
e. Coaches' reports

518. Documentation of caseload, program accomplishments, and summaries comprise the
a. annual report.
b. evaluation records.
c. accreditation reports.
d. filing system.
e. insurance information.

519. OSHA requires records be kept for ____ year (s) if they are for compliance to rules.
a. 1
b. 3
c. 15
d. 30
e. 50

520. How often should general files be reviewed?
a. Annually
b. Biannually
c. Every 5 years
d. Every 7 years
e. Every 10 years

521. The filing system should be set up into
a. separate drawers.
b. separate offices.
c. long-term versus short-term categories.
d. urgent versus short term categories.
e. primary, secondary and tertiary categories.

522. Files that must be kept in locked cabinets include
- a. salary records and budget reports.
- b. medical records and personnel files.
- c. employee contracts and ordering information.
- d. coaches' reports and medical authorizations.
- e. performance evaluation and request for proposals.

523. The accrediting agency for clinics is the
- a. Joint Review Commission.
- b. National Athletic Trainers' Association.
- c. Joint Commission on Accreditation of Healthcare Organizations.
- d. American Physical Therapy Association.
- e. National Collegiate Athletic Association.

524. Which of the following is a policy?
- a. Injury prevention is critical to the safety of athletes.
- b. Pioneer High School will provide athletic trainers for all athletic practices.
- c. Athletic trainers must complete injury reports by the end of each day.
- d. Athletic trainers are to wear polo shirts with the clinic logo.
- e. Employees who take days off are required to find their own replacement.

525. The time in which a person is granted power and authority in a new position is referred to as
- a. the honeymoon effect.
- b. transactional leadership.
- c. personal power.
- d. counterpower.
- e. competency.

526. The role an athletic trainer plays in which there is controlled change is known as
- a. decisional.
- b. entrepreneurial.
- c. disturbance.
- d. influencer.
- e. liaison.

527. What instrument is used to analyze data from various groups of people as the final stage of the strategic planning process?
- a. Analysis of injury statistics
- b. Meyers-Briggs testing
- c. Program evaluation and review technique
- d. Summative evaluation
- e. WOTS UP analysis

528. How long should documentation of mental health records be kept before it is destroyed?
- a. As soon as athlete leaves program
- b. Until athlete is 21years of age
- c. 15 years
- d. 30 years
- e. The life of the individual

529. When mental health records are no longer needed the athletic trainer should

a. throw them in the trash.
b. send them to the athlete.
c. burn them.
d. give them to whomever wants them.
e. put them on microfilm.

530. When can the family of a 21-year-old be informed of his mental health status?
a. When he is unconscious
b. When he is returned to competition
c. When the illness is seven years in duration
d. When he signs an informed consent
e. Whenever the athletic trainer decides to tell them

531. If an attorney calls and requests information regarding an athlete's injury, the athletic trainer should
a. give the attorney all the information he desires.
b. record the conversation on tape.
c. make sure there is an authorized release of information on file first.
d. record the conversation via documentation.
e. refer the attorney to the athlete.

532. For people using whirlpools and sinks to be safe from electrical shock, the national Electric Code requires
a. rubber or tennis shoes.
b. three-pronged plugs.
c. two-pronged plugs.
d. ground-fault interrupters.
e. circuit breaker boxes.

533. An adult athlete does not want his medical condition shared with the coaching staff. When the coach asks for information the best response is
a. "No information can be shared."
b. "I'll get it for you later."
c. "You'll have to ask the athlete's parents."
d. "He is not ready to play."
e. "He is suicidal and needs a referral."

534. The code system used to describe a condition that is put on insurance forms is known as
a. third-party reimbursement.
b. usual customary and reasonable (UCR).
c. explanation of benefits (EOB).
d. current procedural terminology (CPT).
e. international classification of diseases (ICD).

535. An athletic trainer who spends a greater portion than most certified athletic trainers counseling should investigate the code of ethics of the
a. NATA and the NATABOC.
b. American Medical Association and the American Counseling Association.
c. American Medical Association and the NATA.
d. American Counseling Association and the

American Psychological Association.
   e. American Medical Association and the American Physical Therapy Association.

536. Motivation of employees is based on
   a. management style, economics, attitude, and evaluation.
   b. management style, staff development, compensation, and goals.
   c. production, encouragement, supervision, and appreciation.
   d. need, opportunity, ability, and reinforcement.
   e. support, leadership, goals, and management skill.

537. Groups that perform well have administrators who are
   a. task oriented.
   b. employee oriented.
   c. achievement oriented.
   d. constantly rewarding employees.
   e. highly social.

538. Effective performance evaluations must include
   a. trust, all levels of organization, criteria, and rewards for meeting criteria.
   b. knowing who will evaluate strengths and weaknesses.
   c. critical thinking, evaluation of intrinsic and extrinsic factors, and compensation for good evaluation.
   d. learning experiences, success on the job, absenteeism, and power.
   e. ability to delegate, feedback, self-control, and interpersonal relationships.

539. Signs and symptoms of burnout for an athletic trainer include
   a. inability to get ahead, a feeling of closeness, and excitement.
   b. long hours, drug use, and flexibility in hours worked.
   c. headaches, ulcers, and contentment.
   d. fatigue, sleeplessness, depression, and paranoia.
   e. feelings of hopelessness, quitting previous jobs, and high blood pressure.

540. To prevent burnout the athletic trainer should
   a. eat more sugar, exercise regularly, and have outside interests.
   b. take a vacation, manage time, and exercise less.
   c. do more work, do higher quality work, and drink alcohol.
   d. work longer hours, take more vacations, and socialize more.
   e. have realistic goals, exercise regularly, and eat properly.

541. Organizational and administrative tasks of the athletic trainer include

a. education, counseling, rehabilitation, and budgeting.
b. prevention, recognition and evaluation, rehabilitation, and professional development.
c. supervision of staff, education of students, evaluation, and counseling.
d. supervision, policies and procedures, record keeping, and ordering equipment and supplies.
e. research, prevention, immediate care, and rehabilitation.

542. What is the role of the athletic trainer in counseling an athlete?
a. Problem solving for a psychological issue
b. Perform long-term counseling
c. Skill training for a psychological issue
d. Determining possible medication for a psychological issue
e. Treatment planning for a psychological issue

543. The athletic director has instructed you to find insurance to protect the athletic department against medical claims in excess of $50,000. What type of insurance are you in need of?
a. Disability insurance
b. Malpractice insurance
c. Catastrophic insurance
d. Athletic accident insurance
e. Self insurance

544. When referring an athlete for counseling the athletic trainer should consider
a. fee scale and type of counseling required.
b. sex of counselor and availability.
c. ethnicity of counselor and broad-based expertise.
d. age of counselor and comfort level of athlete.
e. expertise of counselor and rapidity to solution of issue.

545. A budget that requires an explanation for each expense made is known as
a. zero-based budgeting.
b. variable budgeting.
c. lump sum budgeting.
d. line-item budgeting.
e. performance budgeting.

546. The purpose of a mission statement is
a. to describe the goals for each employee to aspire.
b. to define policy and procedures.
c. to define organizational philosophy.
d. to assist in decision-making process.
e. to project long- and short-term goals.

547. Strategic plans to be effective must involve
a. the athletic training staff.
b. the students.
c. the administration.
d. the coaches.
e. staff, students, athletes, coaches, and administration.

548. Budgets are to be reviewed
   a. annually.
   b. every 3 years.
   c. every 5 years.
   d. every 7 years.
   e. every 10 years.

■ *Professional Development and Responsibility*

Directions: Each of the questions or incomplete statements here is followed by five suggested answers or completions. Select the best answer in each case.

549. To ensure that questions used in an interview are not discriminatory, avoid questions regarding
   a. previous salary.
   b. benefits desired.
   c. benefactor.
   d. honors and awards.
   e. religion.

550. The NATA Code of Ethics main goal is
   a. to provide the responsibilities of the athletic trainer.
   b. quality health care.
   c. membership services.
   d. limitations of athletic training.
   e. to define standards of practice.

551. The NATA Code of Ethics protects the rights of athletes by
   a. limiting hours worked by the athletic trainer.
   b. limiting services provided by an athletic trainer.
   c. providing scope of practice.
   d. preserving confidentially.
   e. providing level of education for athletic trainers.

552. The NATA Code of Ethics requires that member refrains from
   a. swearing.
   b. substance abuse.
   c. identifying illegal activities.
   d. obtaining parallel credentials.
   e. sex with coaching staff.

553. A member who misrepresents his credentials is in violation of the NATA
   a. mission statement.
   b. continuing education standards.
   c. confidentiality statement.
   d. by-laws.
   e. code of ethics.

554. A member who evaluates an athletic trainer's performance should allow the athletic trainer to review the evaluation or is in violation of the NATA
   a. mission statement.
   b. continuing education standards.
   c. confidentiality statement.
   d. by-laws.
   e. code of ethics.

555. Using the NATA logo as an endorsement for your clinic
   a. is okay.
   b. requires permission of the executive director.

c. is a violation of the NATA mission statement.
d. is a violation of the NATA code of ethics.
e. is a violation of educational requirements.

556. An athletic trainer who receives personal direct money above and beyond his salary from a patient is
a. fortunate.
b. in violation of the code of ethics.
c. charismatic.
d. ethical
e. frugal.

557. The total continuing education credits necessary during a three-year term for a certified athletic trainer is
a. 150.
b. 90.
c. 80.
d. 50.
e. 30.

558. The number of contact hours necessary to equal one continuing education credit is
a. 1.
b. 3.
c. 5.
d. 10.
e. 20.

559. The one ongoing requirement for recertification is
a. first aid.
b. CPR.
c. signing the code of ethics.
d. authoring an article.
e. being a speaker.

560. Upon completion of continuing education requirements the NATABOC will audit
a. all certified athletic trainers.
b. all student certified athletic trainers.
c. randomly all certified athletic trainers.
d. only those with CEU problems.
e. newly certified athletic trainers.

561. In a high school setting, an athletic trainer will have to prove ____ ____ to retain his job.
a. cost effectiveness
b. financial reimbursement
c. insurance costs
d. contact time
e. financial gain

562. If a certified athletic trainer takes an athletic training course worth three credit hours, it is worth how many NATABOC CEUS?
a. 3.0
b. 1.5
c. 1.0
d. .6
e. .8

563. If a certified athletic trainer attends a clinical symposium which is intended to be used for CEUS, attendance is proven by
a. writing a paper.
b. provide a canceled check.
c. provide a copy of his grade.

d. provide a letter of attendance.
e. provide a copy of brochure.

564. The proof necessary for CPR continuing education credit is
a. letter from the instructor.
b. copy of final test.
c. copy of the card.
d. passing a practical test for another athletic trainer.
e. letter of attendance.

565. If a student becomes certified in the final year of the three-year continuing education cycle, how many CEUS does the student need to obtain that year?
a. 100
b. 80
c. 5.5
d. 2.5
e. 0

566. The certified athletic trainer is required to maintain the continuing education file for _____ year(s) after a reporting period.
a. 7
b. 5
c. 3
d. 2
e. 1

567. If an athletic trainer has more CEUS in the three-year period than is required, the CEUS are
a. carried over into the next three-year term.
b. half are carried over into the next three-year term.
c. only publication CEUs are carried over into the next three-year term.
d. only college course CEUs are carried over into the next three-year term.
e. unusable.

568. The Approved Provider Directory is
a. a list of the only providers to be used for CEUS.
b. a list of the only providers that provide quality CEUS.
c. a list of the only providers that provide names of continuing education courses.
d. a list of the only courses reviewed for quality by the Board of Directors.
e. a list of the only courses run by certified athletic trainers.

569. Nonpayment of membership dues can result in
a. suspension of certification.
b. increase of annual dues for all certified members.
c. increase in annual dues for all members.
d. increase in annual dues for all noncertified members.
e. increase CEU and fees for reinstatement.

570. If a certified athletic trainer takes an English class for three college credit hours, it's worth _____ NATABOC CEUS.
a. 9
b. 6
c. 3
d. 1
e. 0

571. How many performance domains are there in athletic training as acknowledged by the NATA?
a. 4
b. 5
c. 6
d. 8
e. 10

572. A recently certified athletic trainer who has two years left in the three year CEU cycle is required to have
a. 80 CEUs.
b. 55 CEUs.
c. 25 CEUs.
d. 5.5 CEUs.
e. 0 CEUs.

573. Occupational Safety and Health Administration's (OSHA) standards for bloodborne pathogens requires records not put into an employee's file must be kept for
a. 1 year.
b. 3 years.
c. 7 years.
d. 15 years.
e. 30 years.

574. The components of negligence include
a. tort, abandonment, government immunity, liability, and risk.
b. informed consent, foreseeability, product failure, and proximate cause.
c. dangerous treatment, assumption of risk, warning, failure to supervise, and duty.
d. malpractice, immunity, comparative negligence, failure to provide instruction, and liability.
e. breach of duty, damage, causation, conduct, and existence of duty.

575. Information can be disseminated by computer via
a. listserve and video conference.
b. the Web and conference calls.
c. pamphlets and software.
d. network and bulletin boards.
e. electronic mail and educational seminars.

576. When evaluating the success of a public relations plan in a clinical setting, it is critical to
a. dress nicely.
b. speak professionally.
c. advertise in many places.
d. spend a lot of money.
e. get feedback from patients.

577. The Fair Labor Standards Act is designed to
a. determine a reasonable workweek.
b. determine insurance coverage.
c. determine death benefits.
d. determine quality of care.
e. determine salary of workers.

578. The purpose of the NATABOC Approved Provider Program is
a. to raise money for the NATA.
b. to provide a network that is easily accessible for the athletic trainer.

c. to raise money for the approved providers.
d. to encourage development of educational programs.
e. to provide strong educational programs for athletic trainers.

579. Sexual harassment by an athletic trainer toward another athletic trainer is
a. not illegal.
b. a breach of the NATA Code of Ethics.
c. just between friends.
d. inappropriate yet sometimes understandable.
e. based on the harasser's point of view.

580. The athletic trainer should project a ____ presence.
a. know-it-all
b. calm
c. informed
d. anxious
e. dominating

581. When designing a brochure with information about the field of athletic training, it should answer
a. how much pay is necessary.
b. benefits and fringe benefits required.
c. expectations and policies of an athletic trainer.
d. years of experience and training.
e. who we are, when we serve, where we work, why we are needed, and how we help.

582. Usual, customary, and reasonable fees are based on
a. the fee requested by a particular clinic.
b. the fee requested by a particular clinic, but the insurance company pays the average amount for that injury based on national statistics for request.
c. the normal fee for a particular service, in a particular area, whichever is lower.
d. the normal fee for a particular medical person for a particular injury.
e. the normal fee for a particular injury.

583. States with very few athletic trainers often are covered by which form of state regulation?
a. Licensure
b. Registration
c. Certification
d. Exemption
e. Board of review

584. While working in a collegiate setting, the student athletic trainer should protect herself against legal action by having
a. good health insurance.
b. malpractice and liability insurance.
c. athletic benefit insurance.
d. catastrophic insurance.
e. a good connection with the boss.

585. What is the general statute of limitations for adults when filing a negligence claim?
a. 1 year
b. 3 years
c. 5 years
d. 7 years
e. 10 years

586. If a minor wants to file a lawsuit for negligence, what is the general statue of limitations?
a. 3 years
b. 3 years after the age of 18
c. 5 years after the age of 18
d. 10 years after the age of 18
e. Indefinitely

587. The agency that enforces regulations on anabolic steroids is the
a. Food and Drug Administration (FDA).
b. Drug Enforcement Authority (DEA).
c. State Board of Pharmacy.
d. State Board of Medicine.
e. Office of Physician Regulation.

588. Drugs that may be abused are enforced by what agency?
a. Food and Drug Administration (FDA).
b. Drug Enforcement Authority (DEA).
c. State Board of Pharmacy.
d. State Board of Medicine.
e. Office of Physician Regulation.

589. The NCAA mandates drug testing at the collegiate level to
a. keep track of substance abusers.
b. keep track of substances used by athletes.
c. assist the United States Olympic Committee (USOC) in determining whom to test.
d. increase revenue.
e. ensure equitable competition.

590. If a college athlete tests positive for the first time for a banned substance, he or she is restricted from competition by the NCAA
a. until there is a negative drug test.
b. for one year.
c. for one season.
d. for one year with negative drug test during that year.
e. indefinitely, pending litigation.

591. Which of the following can cause revocation of certification by the NATABOC?
a. A traffic violation
b. No paying NATA dues on time
c. Being guilty of a misdemeanor related to health care of an athlete
d. Being found not guilty of a misdemeanor related to health care of an athlete
e. By not getting enough CEUs in a 3-year period

592. An athlete with AIDS can participate in sports because AIDS is viewed as a

a. disease by the National Center of Study on Sudden Death.
b. disease by the World Health Organization.
c. virus by the U.S. Department of Education.
d. disability by the Americans With Disability Act.
e. disadvantage by OSHA.

593. If an athlete tests positive for a banned substance a second time, the penalty from the NCAA is

a. one year of eligibility from previous and this year's calendar year of competition.
b. one season of eligibility.
c. indefinitely.
d. this season of competition but may compete in other sports.
e. two years.

594. The World Health Organization guidelines on athletes with HIV indicate

a. no participation can occur.
b. no participation in contact sports.
c. no participation in collision sports.
d. all athletes should be tested.
e. cleaning and covering of bleeding wounds must be done.

595. To prevent athletic department financial loss due to injury, the athletic trainer should review injury statistics. Another term for this is

a. liability.
b. malpractice.
c. misfeasance.
d. duty.
e. risk management.

596. Blank lines in a chart between dated entries

a. are unacceptable.
b. makes the chart look more professional.
c. leaves room for additional information, as needed later.
d. is proper documentation etiquette.
e. needs to be filled in before the patient is released.

597. The most respected test for drugs is

a. the athlete is saying they have or have not used drugs.
b. previous health history.
c. a blood test.
d. enzyme multiplied immunoassay technique.
e. gas chromatography-mass spectrometry.

598. In a high school setting, the employment of an athletic trainer for the first time will

a. increase costs for the school system.
b. decrease costs for the school system.
c. keep costs about the same for the school system.
d. decrease health care.
e. increase liability risk.

599. When asking an athlete about substance abuse, the questions should be

a. straightforward.
b. asked directly.
c. nonjudgmental.
d. intimidating.
e. written down and documented.

600. Which of the following is a legal question in an interview?

a. How many children do you have?
b. How many years have you been married?
c. What illnesses do you have?
d. What physical disabilities do you have?
e. Is weekend work okay for you?

CHAPTER

Study Questions for the Practical Test

The following situations are given to simulate the practical examination. During this portion of the examination you will have an opportunity to demonstrate your skills. These situations are ones with which an entry-level certified athletic trainer will be faced on a daily basis. The examiner's evaluation is based only on your demonstrations to the specific question asked. A model will be the person upon whom you will demonstrate your skills. There will be materials available for your use. But if there is some item you would normally use that is not available, then tell the examiners. The model does not answer your questions and will only do those things you direct them to do.

In this section your goal is to obtain as many positive responses as you can. Questions in this area range from acute injuries, equipment fitting, taping and wrapping, rehabilitation, and management of life-threatening injuries.

You will need another person to assist you in this chapter by reading the questions and checking yes or no for correct and incorrect responses. You will also need a volunteer to be the model. You can follow along in this study guide as your selected examiner reads the questions from Appendix B. The selected examiner can tell you if you have passed a certain oral/practical question, as I have listed a 70% passing point range at the end of each question in Appendix B.

1. Application of Skin Closures. This situation will allow you an opportunity to demonstrate application of skin closures to a wound on the forearm. You will have three minutes to complete your task. Supplies: skin closures, tincture of benzoin, and latex gloves.

2. Assessing Breath Sounds. This situation will allow you to demonstrate assessing breath sounds. Please use the stethoscope to assess breathing. You will have five minutes to complete this task. Supplies: stethoscope.

3. **Use of a Sling Psychrometer.** This situation gives you an opportunity to demonstrate the use of a sling psychrometer to measure the heat index. You will have five minutes to complete your task. Supplies: sling psychrometer and a bowl of water.

4. **Vision Screening.** This situation will allow you to demonstrate the use of a Snellen eye chart. You will have five minutes to complete your task. Supplies: Snellen eye chart mounted on the wall, measuring tape mounted on floor, and an index card.

5. **Limb Girth Measurement.** This situation will allow you to demonstrate limb girth of the knee post surgical to determine atrophy. You will have five minutes to complete your task. Supplies: two measuring tapes.

6. **Postural Screening.** This situation will allow you to demonstrate a standing postural screening laterally. You will have five minutes to complete your task. Supplies: measuring tape, plumb line with plumb bob hanging from ceiling, and a long pole.

7. **Cane Fitting.** This situation will allow you to demonstrate fitting a cane for an athlete with a left lower leg injury. You will have five minutes to complete your task. Supplies: several canes of varying length and a measuring tape.

8. **Deep Reflex Testing.** This situation will allow you to demonstrate the Babinski response. You will have five minutes to complete your task. Supplies: rubber hammer and tongue depressor.

9. **Fitting a Lateral Prophylactic Knee Brace.** This situation will allow you to demonstrate the proper fitting of a lateral hinged prophylactic knee brace. You will have five minutes to complete your task. Supplies: Lateral hinged knee brace with neoprene straps, inch and a half tape, and an elastic bandage.

10. **Use of Otoscope.** This situation will allow you to demonstrate the use of the otoscope for examination of the ear. You will have five minutes to complete your task. Supplies: otoscope and specula.

11. **PNF Contract Relax Stretching.** This situation allows you to perform the contract-relax PNF stretching technique for the hamstring muscle group. You will have five minutes to complete this task. Supplies: supportive padded table.

12. **Single Person Walking Assist.** This situation allows you to perform the removal of an athlete from the field using a walking assist, for an athlete with an injury of the left lower leg. You will have five minutes to complete this task. Supplies: none.

13. Manual Muscle Testing of the Neck. This situation gives you an opportunity to demonstrate manual muscle testing of the neck. You will have five minutes to complete your task. Supplies: none.

14. Use of the Goniometer. This situation gives you an opportunity to demonstrate the range of motion of the second metacarpophalangeal joint using a goniometer. You will have five minutes to complete your task. Supplies: finger goniometer.

15. Testing the Cranial Nerves. This situation gives you an opportunity to test the twelve cranial nerves both motor and sensory. You will have five minutes to complete your task. Supplies: ammonia capsule, Snellen eye chart, spoon, penlight, food, and a paper clip.

16. Hip Adductor Strain Wrapping. Please demonstrate how you would wrap a hip adductor strain. You have three minutes within which to complete your task. Supplies: two-inch adhesive white tape, one and one half-inch adhesive white tape, tape adherent, six-inch elastic bandage, and scissors.

17. Collateral Interphalangeal Joint Taping. This situation gives you an opportunity to tape a finger for instability of the collateral ligaments. You will have three minutes to complete your task. Supplies: scissors, half-inch white adhesive tape.

18. Anterior Drawer Test. This situation gives you an opportunity to demonstrate your ability to perform the anterior drawer test for anterior cruciate ligament instability. You will have five minutes to complete your task. Supplies: none.

19. Apley's Compression Test. This situation gives you an opportunity to demonstrate Apley's compression test of the knee, for assessing a meniscus injury. You will have five minutes to complete your task. Supplies: none.

20. Four-Way Straight Leg Raising. This situation gives you an opportunity to demonstrate four-way straight leg raising exercises for rehabilitation of the lower extremity. You will have five minutes to complete your task. Supplies: none.

21. Thomas Test. The following question gives you an opportunity to demonstrate the Thomas test for determining hip flexor muscle tightness. You will have five minutes to complete your task. Supplies: none.

22. Trendelenburg Test. This situation gives you an opportunity to demonstrate the Trendelenburg test for gluteus medius weakness. You will have five minutes to complete your task. Supplies: none.

23. Codman Pendulum Shoulder Exercises. This situation will allow you to demonstrate Codman pendulum exercises for the shoulder. You will have five minutes to complete your task. Supplies: none.

24. Apprehension Test of the Shoulder. This situation gives you an opportunity to demonstrate the apprehension test to assess instability of the shoulder. You will have five minutes to complete your task. Supplies: none.

25. Range of Motion of the Cervical Spine. This situation gives you an opportunity to demonstrate range of motion of the cervical spine. Muscle testing and neurological testing have been completed. You will have five minutes to complete your task. Supplies: none.

26. Louisiana Ankle Wrap. This situation gives you an opportunity to demonstrate use of Louisiana ankle wrap of the ankle. Please use any of the materials on the table to complete your task. You have three minutes to complete your task.

27. Thumb Check Rein for Hyperextension. This situation gives you an opportunity to tape for thumb hyperextension using the check rein taping technique. You will have three minutes to complete your task. Supplies: tape adherent, scissors, and one and one-half-inch adhesive white tape.

28. Metatarsal Arch Pad Application. This situation gives you an opportunity to apply a pad to the metatarsal arch. Please demonstrate how to apply a pad to the metatarsal arch. You will have three minutes to complete your task. Supplies: half-inch felt, one and one half-inch adhesive white tape, two-inch elastic tape, tape adherent, and scissors.

29. Glenohumeral Glide. This situation will give you an opportunity to demonstrate anterior and posterior glides with distraction of the glenohumeral joint. You will have five minutes to complete your task.

30. Open Basket Weave. This situation gives you the opportunity to tape an acutely injured ankle with an open basket weave and a horseshoe. The athlete has injured the lateral aspect of the ankle. You will have three minutes to complete your task. Supplies: tape adherent, scissors, felt horseshoe (1/2-inch thick), one and one half-inch adhesive white tape, half-inch adhesive white tape, lace and heel pads (with white petroleum jelly), and elastic bandage.

31. Great Toe Sprain Taping. This situation gives you an opportunity to tape a great toe sprain. You will have three minutes to complete your task. Supplies: one half-inch adhesive white tape, tape adherent, elastic tape, pre-wrap, gauze pad, scissors, one and one half-inch tape.

32. **Application of Immobilizer of the Knee (Postinjury).** This situation gives you an opportunity to apply a knee immobilizer to a knee sprain. You will have three minutes to complete your task. Supplies: knee immobilizer.

33. **Hamstring Strain Wrapping.** Please demonstrate how you would wrap a hamstring strain. You have three minutes within which to complete your task. Supplies: two-inch adhesive white tape, one and one half-inch adhesive white tape, tape adherent, white petroleum jelly, pads, six-inch elastic bandage, and scissors.

34. **Knee Pressure Wrapping for Acute Injury.** This situation will allow you an opportunity to demonstrate the skill of pressure wrapping a knee for an acute injury. You will have three minutes to complete your task. Supplies: a double six-inch elastic bandage, one and one-half-inch adhesive white tape, tape adherent, scissors, eight-inch square of felt, and six-inch elastic bandage.

35. **Blister Padding.** This situation gives you an opportunity to demonstrate padding and taping over a closed half-inch sized blister on the ball of the foot. Please use any of the materials on the table to complete your task. You have three minutes to complete your task. Supplies: scissors, quarter-inch foam, adhesive white tape, tape adherent, pre-wrap, first aid cream, Band-Aid, and elastic tape.

36. **Glenohumeral Joint Spica Wrap.** This situation gives you an opportunity to spica wrap the glenohumeral joint for an anterior subluxation. You have three minutes to complete your task. Supplies: double six-inch elastic bandage, two-inch elastic tape, one and one half-inch white tape, and scissors.

37. **Elbow Epicondylitis Taping.** This situation gives you an opportunity to apply tape to a lateral elbow epicondylitis. You will have three minutes to complete your task. Supplies: half-inch felt pad, three-inch elastic tape, pre-wrap, scissors, and one and one-half-inch adhesive white tape.

38. **Acromioclavicular Joint Contusion Padding.** This situation gives you an opportunity to pad the acromioclavicular joint. You will have three minutes to complete your task. Supplies: Band-Aid, half-inch foam padding, tape adherent, one and one half-inch adhesive white tape, scissors, and two-inch elastic tape.

8
CHAPTER

Study Questions for the Written Simulation

The written simulation section in this manual is designed to be similar to the certification examination. In this section of the test you will be tested on your decision-making skills in situations an entry-level certified athletic trainer faces on a daily basis. The actual certification examination uses two booklets, a problem guide, and an answer guide in which you make your responses with a highlight pen. There is a highlight pen used the day you actually take the test. In this manual, I have placed the "highlights" in brackets in Appendix C (page 178). You will need a partner to assist you with this portion of the study test. As you select an answer for each item in a problem, your partner should have Appendix B open and read the "highlight" corresponding to the item you are working on. Based on the information you know from the opening scene, and what you find through answering the questions, select only those answers necessary at that time. You are to read the problem and carefully decide all of the options in each section you would choose for your athlete. Some sections will have more than one appropriate response, so choose all that apply. If you choose an incorrect response, you will receive a penalty. Also, a penalty will be given if you fail to choose all correct responses. As you highlight, answer-specific instructions are given, and you must then follow this information to solve the problem correctly.

Problem 1

Opening Scene: You are told that an athlete has collapsed at the finish line of a cross country race. Today's temperature is 75 degrees F.

A. What is your initial assessment of this situation? (Choose only those actions that you have reason to believe are essential to the resolution of the case at this time.)
   1. Ask the athlete what happened.
   2. Determine what place the person finished.
   3. Determine if the athlete has a pulse.

4. Visually check the athlete's body position.
5. Determine if the athlete is breathing.
6. Determine athlete's level of consciousness.
7. Ask the athlete if there is any pain other than already noted.
8. Ask athlete about her health history.
9. Ask the athlete about pain.
10. Determine skin color.
11. Ask athlete if this injury has happened before.

B. Given the previous information what would you do now to resolve this situation? (Choose only those actions that you have reason to believe are essential to the resolution of the case at this time.)

12. Palpate athlete's ankle.
13. Check the athlete's skin temperature.
14. Smell the athlete's breath.
15. Ask athlete if she is allergic to anything.
16. Ask athlete about her fluid consumption today.
17. Check athlete's pulse rate.
18. Check athlete's breathing rate.
19. Ask about the athlete's last meal eaten.
20. Hold athlete's head.
21. Check the athlete's blood pressure.

C. What is your initial treatment of this injury in this situation? (Choose only those actions that you have reason to believe are essential to the resolution of the case at this time.)

22. Auscultate the chest.
23. Give the athlete a shot of epinephrine solution.
24. Have athlete sit or lie down.
25. Call for the coach.
26. Pour cool water over the athlete.
27. Remove restrictive clothing.
28. Apply ice.
29. Apply a pressure bandage.
30. Check ankle range of motion.
31. Give the athlete an inhaler.
32. Demonstrate the drawer sign.
33. Give the athlete food to eat.
34. Encourage the athlete to breathe into a paper bag.
35. Move everything away from the athlete.
36. Place an object between the athlete's teeth.
37. Give athlete unrestricted fluids by mouth.
38. Give athlete mouth-to-mouth resuscitation.

39. Backboard the athlete.
40. Place athlete on crutches.

D. Given the previous information, what illness or injury has this athlete suffered? Choose only one answer.
41. A collapsed lung.
42. Asthma attack.
43. Insulin shock.
44. Ankle sprain.
45. Dehydration.
46. A bee sting.
47. Hyperglycemia.
48. Hyperventilation.
49. The flu.
50. A seizure.
51. Heat stroke.

E. Given the information you have at this time, what would you do to prevent this situation from reoccurring? (Choose only those actions that you have reason to believe are essential to the resolution of the problem at this time.)
52. Use an inhaler.
53. Have athlete wear chest protector.
54. Empty all trash cans.
55. Have athlete eat periodically.
56. Keep a chart of daily weight loss.
57. Make sure athlete takes seizure medication.
58. Allow unlimited access to water.
59. Have athlete consume water pre-exercise.
60. Have athlete take salt tablets.
61. Have athlete take vitamins.
62. Tape both ankles.
63. Acclimatize the athlete.

Problem 2

Opening Scene: A football running back is lying on the ground after a play. You are waved onto the field by the game official.

A. What is your initial assessment of this situation? (Choose only those actions that you have reason to believe are essential to the resolution of the case at this time.)
1. Ask athlete what happened.
2. Roll the athlete while controlling the head and neck.
3. Determine if the athlete is conscious.
4. Remove athlete's helmet.

5. Check the scene.
6. Remove his mouth guard.
7. Remove face mask.
8. Determine if the athlete has a heartbeat.
9. Ask teammates what happened.
10. Determine if the airway is open.
11. Open airway using chin lift method.
12. Elevate athlete's feet.
13. Determine if the athlete is breathing.
14. Carry athlete off the field.
15. Open the airway using the head tilt method.
16. Call for help.
17. Call for ambulance.

B. Given the previous information what would you do now to resolve this situation? (Choose only those actions that you have reason to believe are essential to the resolution of the problem at this time.)

18. Apply ice to the fracture.
19. Apply a sling and swathe.
20. Palpate the athlete's head and face.
21. Check breathing rate and quality.
22. Straighten fracture.
23. Remove athlete's helmet.
24. Stabilize the athlete's head and neck.
25. Check pulse rate and quality.
26. Pinch the athlete.
27. Have student athletic trainer check emergency medical card.
28. Take blood pressure.
29. Check pupils.
30. Look for severe bleeding.
31. Check for medical alert tag.

C. Given the information you have at this time, what would you do next to resolve this issue? (Choose only those actions that you have reason to believe are essential to the resolution of the problem at this time.)

32. Elevate athlete's feet and arms.
33. Palpate the abdominal quadrants.
34. Palpate cervical spine.
35. Palpate sternum.
36. Palpate both legs.
37. Palpate thoracic spine.
38. Check for referred pain.
39. Palpate both arms.
40. Recheck pulse and breathing.

41. Listen for breath sounds.
42. Palpate the chest.
43. Check body temperature.
44. Palpate hips.
45. Listen for heart sounds.

D. Given the information you have at this time, what would you do next to resolve this issue? (Choose only those actions that you have reason to believe are essential to the resolution of the problem at this time.)

46. Turn athlete onto his side.
47. Remove face mask.
48. Check athlete's airway.
49. Check athlete's breathing.
50. Place sandbags, blanket roll, or commercial head immobilizer.
51. Strap athlete's head to the board.
52. Remove athlete's shoulder pads.
53. Place an open ammonia capsule under the athlete's nose.
54. Place a bite splint between athlete's teeth.
55. Place a rigid neck collar on athlete.
56. Cross chest strap athlete.
57. Check capillary refill.
58. Have the student athletic trainer bring a backboard.
59. Secure athlete's hips to board.
60. Log roll athlete.
61. Have a student athletic trainer available to direct the ambulance.
62. Secure athlete's legs to board.

E. Given the information you have at this time, what would you do next to resolve this issue? (Choose only those actions that you have reason to believe are essential to the resolution of the problem at this time.)

63. Apply direct pressure.
64. Apply air splint.
65. Elevate limb.
66. Elevate athlete's head.
67. Apply pressure bandage.
68. Give athlete glucose in the cheek.
69. Cover athlete with a blanket.
70. Remove athlete from the field
71. Send athlete to hospital.

Problem 3

Opening Scene: You are working a rugby game for the first time with this team. An adult rugby player is lying supine on the field. Once play is stopped you are summoned onto the field.

A. What is your initial assessment of this situation? (Choose only those actions that you have reason to believe are essential to the resolution of the problem at this time.)
   1. Check circulation.
   2. Check airway.
   3. Call for help.
   4. Ask the officials to stop the unnecessary roughness during the game.
   5. Check for bleeding and deformity.
   6. Remove the athlete from the field.
   7. Determine if the scene is safe.
   8. Grab your training kit and run onto the field.
   9. Ask the athlete the specific area of pain.
   10. Determine athlete's level of consciousness.
   11. Give the athlete aspirin.
   12. Determine the jersey number of the athlete who injured your player.
   13. Check for a medical alert tag.
   14. Stabilize her head and neck using both hands.
   15. Ask the athlete what happened.
   16. Check breathing.

B. Given the information you have at this time, what would you do next to resolve this issue? (Choose only those actions that you have reason to believe are essential to the resolution of the problem at this time.)
   17. Determine a blood pressure.
   18. Determine if a family member is around.
   19. Take the pulse.
   20. Walk the athlete off the field.
   21. Insert an airway.
   22. Determine the athlete's level of skill.
   23. Call an ambulance.
   24. Have the athlete sit up.
   25. Have athlete move her legs.
   26. Get your splint kit.
   27. Ask the athlete if she has a history of this same injury.
   28. Determine respiratory rate.
   29. Have the athlete move her arms.
   30. Roll the athlete to determine a back injury.

C. Given the information you have at this time, what would you do next to resolve this issue? (Choose only those actions that you have reason to believe are essential to the resolution of the problem at this time.)

31. Place an ammonia capsule under her nose.
32. Ask the athlete about previous illnesses.
33. Check the athlete's hearing.
34. Ask the athlete about allergies.
35. Perform Romberg test.
36. Have athlete make faces.
37. Have athlete elevate her shoulders.
38. Ask the athlete about current medications.
39. Ask the athlete if the pain is mild, moderate, or severe.
40. Have athlete stick her tongue out.
41. Call for an ambulance.

D. Given the information you have at this time, what would you do next to resolve this issue? (Choose only those actions that you have reason to believe are essential to the resolution of the problem at this time.)

42. Place cool wet towels around the athlete's head and shoulders.
43. Cover the athlete with a blanket.
44. Take the athlete's temperature using the back of your hand.
45. Observe head and face.
46. Ask the athlete if she has been drinking.
47. Check athlete for a wallet.
48. Remove the athlete's uniform.
49. Give the athlete water to drink.
50. Check pupils.
51. Observe throat.
52. Check ears.
53. Palpate each side of neck, without touching cervical spine.
54. Give the athlete some caffeine pills.
55. Palpate scalp.
56. Palpate throat.
57. Check mouth.
58. Check nose.
59. Take the athlete's temperature rectally.
60. Ask athlete when her last meal was.
61. Palpate face.
62. Elevate the athlete's head.
63. Ask athlete if she has ever had a head injury before.
64. Ask athlete to tell you if anything hurts as you touch a part.

E. Given the information you have at this time, what would you do next to resolve this issue? (Choose only those actions that you have reason to believe are essential to the resolution of the problem at this time.)

65. Place a backboard under the athlete.
66. Roll the athlete while stabilizing the head.

67. Recheck vital signs.
68. Have the athlete eat some granular sugar.
69. Give mouth-to-mouth breathing.
70. Strap the legs to the backboard.
71. Tape or strap the athlete's head to the board.
72. Determine the time of injury for documentation.
73. Reassure the athlete.
74. Place the athlete in a cold shower.
75. Cover athlete with a blanket.
76. Place a rigid neck collar on the athlete.
77. Elevate the athlete's feet.
78. Cross chest strap.
79. Begin CPR.
80. Give the athlete a cup of water to drink.

F. Given the information you have, what do you believe is wrong with this athlete? (Choose only those actions that you have reason to believe are essential to the resolution of the problem at this time.)

81. Respiratory arrest.
82. Heat stroke.
83. Heat exhaustion.
84. Diabetic coma.
85. Cardiac arrest.
86. Head injury.
87. Insulin shock.
88. Nothing, athlete is malingering.
89. Spinal cord injury.

G. Given the information you have at this time, what would you advise this athlete to do to prevent this situation again? (Choose only those actions that you have reason to believe are essential to the resolution of the problem at this time.)

90. Eat one to two hours before playing.
91. Seek the advice of a dietician.
92. Wear a helmet.
93. Wear a chest protector.
94. Have the athlete quit playing.
95. Monitor weight before and after practice.
96. Drink plenty of fluids.
97. Wear lightweight clothing.
98. Athlete should wear a mouth guard.
99. Take salt tablets.
100. Check heat and humidity before practice.
101. Eat a well-balanced diet.

102. Give insulin one hour prior to exercise.
103. Eat every 30 minutes of the game.

Problem 4

Opening Scene: Two track athletes run into the training room, indicating an athlete is hurt.

A. What is your initial response to this situation? (Choose only those actions that you have reason to believe are essential to the resolution of the problem at this time.)
   1. Ask for directions to the track.
   2. Call for a parent.
   3. Ask the students the name of the athlete.
   4. Wash your hands.
   5. Grab your training kit.
   6. Call your friends and let them know you are busy.
   7. Run to the track.
   8. Calm the other students down.
   9. Call a custodian to lock the gates on the track.
   10. Ask if they know if the athlete has any previous injuries.
   11. Send the students back to the track to tell the athlete you are on the way.
   12. Find the track coach.
   13. Do not do anything, students usually overreact.
   14. Ask if the athlete is a star on the team.
   15. Grab some ice.
   16. Search for the emergency medical cards.
   17. Lock the door to the training room.

B. Given the information you have at this time, what would you do next to resolve this issue? (Choose only those actions that you have reason to believe are essential to the resolution of the problem at this time.)
   18. Give two full breaths.
   19. Elevate the arms and legs.
   20. Call for help.
   21. Check for a pulse in the neck.
   22. Determine if the scene is safe.
   23. Determine from bystanders what happened.
   24. Check for severe bleeding.
   25. Determine level of consciousness.
   26. Roll the athlete while controlling his head.
   27. Remove constrictive clothing around the neck and waist.
   28. Open airway using chin lift.
   29. Auscultate the chest.

30. Begin a secondary survey.
31. Look, listen, and feel for breathing.
32. Use a one-way pocket face mask.

C. Given the information you have at this time, what would you do next to resolve this issue? (Choose only those actions that you have reason to believe are essential to the resolution of the problem at this time.)

33. Check the throat for a foreign object.
34. Give 8 to 10 Heimlich maneuvers or abdominal thrusts.
35. Give a pre-cardiac thump.
36. Take a blood pressure.
37. Place two fingers upon the lower portion of the sternum.
38. Finger sweep.
39. Blow hard past the object.
40. Feel up the ribs.
41. Slap athlete on the back five times.
42. Roll the athlete prone.
43. Give two full breaths.
44. Press on the abdomen.
45. Remove vomitus.
46. Open airway.
47. Give two full breaths.
48. Roll the athlete onto his side.
49. Reopen airway.
50. Cover the athlete with a blanket.
51. Give 15 compressions.
52. Continue to give Heimlich maneuvers.
53. Continue mouth-to-mouth resuscitation.

D. Given the information you have at this time, what would you do next to resolve this issue? (Choose only those actions that you have reason to believe are essential to the resolution of the problem at this time.)

54. Continue to give Heimlich maneuvers.
55. Check pupils.
56. Give two person mouth-to-mouth resuscitation.
57. Check the body temperature.
58. Check pulse rate.
59. Continue mouth-to-mouth resuscitation.
60. Give two-person cardiopulmonary resuscitation.
61. Check breathing rate.
62. Paramedics arrive, allow paramedics to assume CPR.
63. Check for severe bleeding.
64. Turn athlete on his side.

E. Given the information you have at this time, what would you do next to resolve this issue? (Choose only those actions that you have reason to believe are essential to the resolution of the problem at this time.)
  65. Rope off the area.
  66. Call the school's social worker.
  67. Get a history.
  68. Check the type of insurance the athlete may have.
  69. Check to see if you paid your malpractice insurance.
  70. Read your policy and procedures manual.
  71. Document what happened.
  72. Ask the track coach what happened.
  73. Lock all gates to the track.
  74. Backboard the athlete.
  75. Call the parents.

F. The athletic director indicates the athlete will be fine. What would you do to prevent the injury from occurring to another athlete? (Choose only those actions that you have reason to believe are essential to the resolution of the problem at this time.)
  76. Call the weather to determine if a storm is coming.
  77. Set a policy on severe weather and storms.
  78. Have a policy to who makes the call to remove athletes from field.
  79. Contact the team physician.
  80. Determine safe areas for storms.
  81. Work with the track coach on a conditioning program.
  82. Issue a statement no longer permitting chewing gum while exercising.
  83. Purchase a lightning detector.
  84. Lock the track.
  85. Provide a more in-depth school pre-participation physical.
  86. Set policy on supervision of all athletes.

Problem 5

Opening Scene: You and a student are working in the training room. An athlete staggers into the training room, blood rushing down his face and both arms.

A. What is your initial assessment of this situation? (Choose only those actions that you have reason to believe are essential to the resolution of the problem at this time.)
  1. Determine if athlete is breathing.
  2. Apply latex gloves.
  3. Get several self-adhesive bandage strips.

4. Check airway.
5. Determine hospital needed to give stitches.
6. Give the athlete some gauze.
7. Determine if the scene is safe.
8. Have the student put on latex gloves.
9. Determine when the incident occurred.
10. Determine what happened.
11. Elevate the arms.

B. Given the information you have at this time, what would you do next to resolve this issue? (Choose only those actions that you have reason to believe are essential to the resolution of the problem at this time.)

12. Elevate the athlete's arms.
13. Tell the athlete to throw the ball outside.
14. Have the athlete lie down.
15. Apply direct pressure to his arms.
16. Have student call for an ambulance.
17. Have the athlete sit down.
18. Call the student's name.
19. Do a head to toe assessment of the student.
20. Have student apply direct pressure on a wound.
21. Elevate the athlete's feet.
22. Visually survey the student.
23. Determine the number of stitches.
24. Give the athlete some food.
25. Determine the depth of the wounds.
26. Give the athlete a glass of water.
27. Give the athlete some aspirin.
28. Apply tourniquet.
29. Check the athlete's skin color.

C. Given the information you have at this time, what would you do next to resolve this issue? (Choose only those actions that you have reason to believe are essential to the resolution of the problem at this time.)

30. Have the athlete sit up.
31. Apply ice to student's head.
32. Apply a pressure bandage to athlete's arms.
33. Remove glass from athlete's arm.
34. Clean the blood off the athlete.
35. Remove latex gloves and soiled gauze and place in biohazard container.
36. Apply pressure to the carotid artery.
37. Apply a pressure bandage to athlete's head.
38. Apply pressure to the brachial artery.

39. Clean the blood off the equipment.
40. Cover athlete with a blanket.

D. Given the information you have at this time, what would you do next to resolve this issue? (Choose only those actions that you have reason to believe are essential to the resolution of the problem at this time.)

41. Check breathing of student.
42. Apply a cervical spine collar.
43. Begin mouth-to-mouth breathing.
44. Loosen tight clothing.
45. Check school's liability insurance.
46. Call the student's parents.
47. Tell student he cannot work in the training room.
48. Ask student if he has any medical conditions.
49. Call the athletic director.
50. Record a SOAP note on the athlete.
51. Check airway of student.
52. Move objects away from the student.
53. Check circulation of student.
54. Ask student for history.
55. Recheck the athlete.
56. Give the student some food.
57. Give the student some water.
58. Give the student some electrolyte drink.
59. Splint the fracture.
60. Palpate student's head.
61. Determine student's level of consciousness.
62. Ask the student how he is feeling.

E. Given the information you have at this time, what would you do next to resolve this issue? (Choose only those actions that you have reason to believe are essential to the resolution of the problem at this time.)

63. Straighten fracture.
64. Place in a sling.
65. Begin CPR.
66. Give student granular sugar.
67. Place ice on student's head, neck, and armpits.
68. Elevate student's feet.
69. Cover student with a blanket.
70. Place a fan on high toward the student.
71. Apply ice.
72. Elevate student's head.
73. Turn student on his side.
74. Place a spoon between student's teeth.

F. Given the information you have at this time, what would you do next to resolve this issue? (Choose only those actions that you have reason to believe are essential to the resolution of the problem at this time.)
   75. Give the athlete oxygen.
   76. Apply an air splint.
   77. Place slings on both arms.
   78. Check capillary refill in fingertips.
   79. Check athlete's blood pressure.
   80. Check pupil response.
   81. Take athlete's pulse rate.

G. The ambulance arrives. Given the information you have at this time, what would you do next to resolve this issue? (Choose only those actions that you have reason to believe are essential to the resolution of the problem at this time.)
   82. Give paramedics athlete's hospital of choice.
   83. Let them take the athlete to hospital.
   84. Close the training room.
   85. Give medical information.
   86. Let paramedics take the student to hospital.
   87. Call athlete's parents.
   88. Take a depressant.
   89. Drink a cup of coffee to calm down.
   90. Call student's parents.
   91. Document the athlete's injury.
   92. Ride with the athlete.
   93. Document the student's injury
   94. Post a job for more student assistance.

Problem 6

Opening Scene: You are called to the scene in which an athlete is lying on the floor in the locker room.

A. What is your initial assessment of this situation? (Choose only those actions that you have reason to believe are essential to the resolution of the problem at this time.)
   1. Grab your training kit.
   2. Find out who is supervising the locker room.
   3. Shake the athlete vigorously.
   4. Determine what team the athlete is on.
   5. Check scene for safety.
   6. Call for an ambulance.
   7. Determine athlete's level of consciousness.
   8. Ask if anyone saw what happened.

9. Check circulation.
10. Determine which locker belongs to this athlete.
11. Determine which duffel bag belongs to the athlete.
12. Open airway.
13. Check for deformity.
14. Get a combination to the lock on athlete's locker.
15. Look, listen, and feel for breathing.
16. Check for severe bleeding.
17. Run to scene.

B. Given the information you have at this time, what would you do next to resolve this issue? (Choose only those actions that you have reason to believe are essential to the resolution of the problem at this time.)
18. Check airway.
19. Take the pulse.
20. Check breathing.
21. Do urine test for drugs.
22. Determine a blood pressure.
23. Check skin color.
24. Check circulation in the brachial artery.
25. Look for drug paraphernalia.
26. Determine parents' phone number.
27. Determine who is the athlete's coach.
28. Determine respiratory rate.
29. Roll the athlete over.
30. Check pupils for size, equality, and reaction.
31. Check arms for track marks.

C. Given the information you have at this time, what would you do next to resolve this issue? (Choose only those actions that you have reason to believe are essential to the resolution of the problem at this time.)
32. Palpate throat.
33. Give the athlete something to eat.
34. Give the athlete something to drink.
35. Recheck breathing and circulation.
36. Determine the athlete's blood sugar level.
37. Loosen tight clothing.
38. Check mouth.
39. Turn off all phones.
40. Call custodial crew.
41. Call gas company.
42. Palpate scalp.
43. Check area for gas leak.
44. Palpate face.

45. Place athlete on her side.
46. Palpate cervical spine.
47. Cover your face with a mask.
48. Check nose.
49. Drag athlete into the hallway.
50. Visualize neck and throat.

D. Given the information you have at this time, what would you do next to resolve this issue? (Choose only those actions that you have reason to believe are essential to the resolution of the problem at this time.)

51. Palpate the thoracic spine.
52. Visualize the chest for wounds.
53. Recheck breathing and circulation.
54. Palpate the clavicles.
55. Pull fire alarm.
56. Palpate the ribs.
57. Palpate the sternum.
58. Apply direct pressure.
59. Auscultate chest.

E. Given the information you have at this time, what would you do next to resolve this issue? (Choose only those actions that you have reason to believe are essential to the resolution of the problem at this time.)

60. Palpate the upper left quadrant.
61. Apple pressure to a pressure point.
62. Visualize the abdomen and hips.
63. Palpate the lower left quadrant.
64. Start praying.
65. Place sterile dressing over the wound.
66. Auscultate the abdomen.
67. Elevate limb.
68. Palpate the upper right quadrant.
69. Strap limb to the body for additional support.
70. Splint fracture.
71. Palpate the lower right quadrant.
72. Recheck pulse.
73. Apply vacuum splint to limb to control bleeding.
74. Place athlete on backboard.
75. Recheck breathing.
76. Roll athlete.
77. Palpate lumbar spine.

F. Given the information you have at this time, what would you do next to resolve this issue? (Choose only those actions that you have reason to believe are essential to the resolution of the problem at this time.)

78. Place sand bags or blanket around side of head.
79. Control athlete's head.
80. Send someone to get a backboard.
81. Cross chest strap the athlete.
82. Strap athlete's hips.
83. Palpate hips.
84. Go and get a backboard yourself.
85. Recheck breathing and pulse.
86. Palpate right lower extremity.
87. Check capillary refill.
88. Strap the athlete's hands.
89. Palpate left lower extremity.
90. Strap athlete's arms.
91. Place a neck collar on athlete.
92. Visualize both legs.
93. Strap head to the board.
94. Check pulse in posterior tibialis and dorsalis pedis.
95. Elevate the head.
96. Cover athlete with blanket.
97. Perform Babinski test.
98. Elevate feet.

G. Given the information you have at this time, what would you do next to resolve this issue? (Choose only those actions that you have reason to believe are essential to the resolution of the problem at this time.)

99. Palpate the left arm.
100. Check capillary refill.
101. Check radial pulse.
102. Elevate arms.
103. Visualize both arms.
104. Palpate the right arm.
105. Monitor breathing.
106. Monitor heartbeat.

H. The ambulance arrives. What would you do next to resolve this issue? (Choose only those actions that you have reason to believe are essential to the resolution of the problem at this time.)

107. Send athlete via ambulance to hospital.
108. Give the emergency medical technicians vital signs.
109. Phone the parents.
110. Give emergency medical technicians an emergency card with permission to treat.

111. Check surveillance cameras to determine the cause of illness.
112. Open windows to allow fresh air.

Problem 7

Opening Scene: An athlete hops into the training room without placing pressure on one of her legs.

A. What is your initial assessment of this situation? (Choose only those actions that you have reason to believe are essential to the resolution of the problem at this time.)

1. Survey the scene.
2. Determine the athlete's body position.
3. Ask the athlete what happened.
4. Determine if the scene is safe.
5. Ask about previous injuries.
6. Ask where was the pain initially.
7. Determine athlete's level of consciousness.
8. Ask when did injury happen.
9. Spine airway.
10. Ask if she has injured this ankle before.
11. Ask if she continued to play.
12. Determine athlete's breathing rate.
13. Ask if athlete heard or felt a pop, snap, crack, slip, or give.
14. Check carotid for circulation.
15. Check for severe bleeding.
16. Ask if the ankle feels unstable.
17. Determine breathing rate.

B. Given the information you have at this time, what would you do next to resolve this issue? (Choose only those actions that you have reason to believe are essential to the resolution of the problem at this time.)

18. Determine if athlete pronates.
19. Check for tibial varus.
20. Determine if the athlete supinates.
21. Walking gait.
22. Look for toeing in and out.
23. Look for swelling.
24. Check for tibial valgus.
25. Check athlete for pes cavus.
26. Look for deformity.
27. Check for discoloration.
28. Check athlete for pes planus.

C. Given the information you have at this time, what would you do next to resolve this issue? (Choose only those actions that you have reason to believe are essential to the resolution of the problem at this time.)

29. Palpate the interosseous membrane.
30. Check for scars.
31. Palpate the base of the fifth metatarsal.
32. Palpate the calcaneofibular ligament.
33. Palpate the bifurcated ligament.
34. Palpate the ASIS.
35. Palpate the anterior talofibular ligament.
36. Palpate the extensor digitorum longus.
37. Palpate posterior talofibular ligament and peroneal tendons.
38. Palpate the navicular.
39. Palpate the Achilles tendon.
40. Palpate the flexor hallicus longus.
41. Palpate first through fourth metatarsals.
42. Palpate the flexor digitorum longus.
43. Palpate the anterior tibiofibular ligament.
44. Palpate deltoid.
45. Palpate the neck of the fibula.
46. Palpate the femoral artery.
47. Palpate the extensor hallicus longus.
48. Squeeze the mid-shaft of the fibula.
49. Palpate posterior tibialis.
50. Palpate the anterior tibialis.
51. Palpate cuboids.
52. Palpate the inguinal ligament.
53. Palpate phalanges.
54. Palpate medial melleolus.
55. Palpate the sciatic notch.
56. Palpate the lymph nodes.

D. Given the information you have at this time, what would you do next to resolve this issue? (Choose only those actions that you have reason to believe are essential to the resolution of the problem at this time.)

57. Perform distraction test.
58. Apply ice.
59. Check skin temperature.
60. Check calcaneal bursa.
61. Check retrocalcaneal bursa.
62. Check capillary refill.
63. Check greater trochanteric bursa.
64. Check posterior tibial artery.
65. Check dorsal pedal artery.

E. Given the information you have at this time, what would you do next to resolve this issue? (Choose only those actions that you have reason to believe are essential to the resolution of the problem at this time.)
   66. Perform Thompson test.
   67. Have athlete perform active resistive range of motion.
   68. Perform stork standing test.
   69. Perform Thomas test.
   70. Have athlete perform active range of motion.
   71. Perform Gaenslen's Sign.
   72. Perform passive range of motion.
   73. Perform inversion stress test.
   74. Check side-to-side movement of the talus.
   75. Perform Homans' sign.
   76. Perform heel pound test.
   77. Perform anterior drawer test.
   78. Check neurological sensations.
   79. Perform eversion stress test.

F. Given the information you have at this time, what would you do next to resolve this issue? (Choose only those actions that you have reason to believe are essential to the resolution of the problem at this time.)
   80. Place athlete in cold whirlpool.
   81. Begin cryotherapy.
   82. Place athlete on crutches.
   83. Begin petrissage.
   84. Apply analgesic pack.
   85. Apply a horseshoe.
   86. Apple a hot pack.
   87. Elevate leg.

Problem 8

Opening Scene: A baseball player indicates he has a lump on his lip.

A. What is your initial assessment of this situation? (Choose only those actions that you have reason to believe are essential to the resolution of the problem at this time.)
   1. Ask how did it happen.
   2. Ask when did it happen.
   3. Ask where was the pain initially.
   4. Ask have you injured your head before.
   5. Ask do you have a headache.
   6. Ask were you able to continue participating.
   7. Ask the athlete about recent events to determine retrograde amnesia or anterograde amnesia.

8. Ask do you have ringing (tinnitus) in your ears.
9. Ask do you have pain anywhere.
10. Ask what treatment was given initially.
11. Ask who gave the treatment initially.
12. Ask did you lose consciousness.
13. Ask do you feel nauseous or want to vomit.
14. Ask did athlete have a seizure.
15. Ask any weakness or numbness.
16. Ask do you have blurred vision.
17. Ask if he has difficulty swallowing.
18. Ask if he has bouts of hoarseness.
19. Ask athlete if he has been sick lately.
20. Ask if athlete uses any drugs.

B. Given the information you have at this time, what would you do next to resolve this issue? (Choose only those actions that you have reason to believe are essential to the resolution of the problem at this time.)
21. Check skin color.
22. Check for swelling.
23. Check for difficulty speaking.
24. Check pupil symmetry and size.
25. Check eye movements.
26. Check breathing pattern and rate.
27. Check for bleeding, or discoloration about face.
28. Check ability to concentrate.
29. Check for battle sign.
30. Check for leakage of cerebrospinal fluid.
31. Check position of head and neck.
32. Check teeth.
33. Check movement of arms and legs.
34. Check athlete's mouth.
35. Ask athlete if he uses tobacco.
36. Check level of consciousness.

C. Given the information you have at this time, what would you do next to resolve this issue? (Choose only those actions that you have reason to believe are essential to the resolution of the problem at this time.)
37. Palpate frontal bone.
38. Palpate nasal bone.
39. Palpate orbital bone.
40. Palpate mastoid process.
41. Palpate parietal bones.
42. Palpate temporal bones.

43. Palpate zygomatic.
44. Palpate maxilla.
45. Palpate mandible.
46. Palpate neck.
47. Palpate throat.
48. Check lymph nodes.
49. Palpate occipital bone.
50. Palpate ears.

D. Given the information you have at this time, what would you do next to resolve this issue? (Choose only those actions that you have reason to believe are essential to the resolution of the problem at this time.)

51. Check body temperature.
52. Give a Snellen test.
53. Determine skin temperature.
54. Perform Romberg's test.
55. Check blood pressure.
56. Perform finger/nose coordination test.
57. Check for papilledema.
58. Perform pursuit test.
59. Check papillary response.
60. Determine if athlete can purse his lips.

E. Given the information you have at this time, what care would you recommend for this athlete? (Choose only those actions that you have reason to believe are essential to the resolution of the problem at this time.)

61. Refer to physician.
62. Ice.
63. Check the baseball helmet.
64. Wear a mouth guard.
65. Wear sunglasses.
66. Wear a throat protector.
67. Stop using chewing tobacco.
68. Gargle.
69. Take antibiotics.
70. Take aspirin.
71. Apply compression.
72. Rest.

Problem 9

Opening Scene: A teary-eyed coach comes into the training room, blood on his shirt, and wants to talk with you privately.

A. What type of information would you include for employees in this situation? (Choose only those actions that you have reason to believe are essential to the resolution of the problem at this time.)
   1. Pull emergency card.
   2. Reassure the coach.
   3. Ask what injuries the athlete incurred.
   4. Ask the coach whose blood is on his shirt.
   5. Ask coach what he is concerned about.
   6. Ask how the athlete got hurt.
   7. Determine if the athlete is OK.
   8. Ask coach what happened.
   9. Grab training kit and go to track.

B. Given the information you have at this time, what would you do next to resolve this issue? (Choose only those actions that you have reason to believe are essential to the resolution of the problem at this time.)
   10. Refer coach for a blood test.
   11. Have the coach wash his hands.
   12. Put on latex gloves.
   13. Have coach apply his own latex gloves.
   14. Have coach bandage wound.
   15. Dispose of soiled clothing.
   16. Have coach wash his face.
   17. Remove soiled clothing.
   18. Have coach apply antiseptic to wound.
   19. You wash your hands.
   20. Put on face mask and gown.
   21. Place plastic on treatment table before coach sits down.

C. Given the information you have at this time, what would you do next to resolve this issue? (Choose only those actions that you have reason to believe are essential to the resolution of the problem at this time.)
   22. Look over the athlete's history.
   23. Sanitize the sink.
   24. Get a blood test for yourself.
   25. Sanitize with bleach all areas, the coach may have touched.
   26. Dispose of all soiled materials in hazardous materials container.
   27. Place yellow tape around area where coach touched.
   28. Make sure your hepatitis vaccine is up to date.
   29. Increase ventilation in the room.
   30. Increase temperature in the room to kill germs.

D. Given the information you have at this time, what would you do to document this exposure? (Choose only those actions that you have reason to believe are essential to the resolution of the problem at this time.)

31. Treatment of coach.
32. Source of exposure.
33. Coach's medical history prior to this exposure.
34. Counseling provided.
35. Coach's state of mind.
36. Time of day.
37. Determine if source will give permission for a blood sample.
38. Prevention of reoccurrence.
39. When exposure occurred.
40. Place where exposure occurred.
41. Protection used.
42. Means of exposure.
43. Witnesses to the exposure.

E. The athletic director has asked you to develop a program to manage blood-borne pathogens. Given the information you have at this time, what would you do next to resolve this issue? (Choose only those actions that you have reason to believe are essential to the resolution of the problem at this time.)

44. Modes of transmission.
45. How to report an exposure.
46. Informing student-athletes and parents of the risk.
47. Types of protective equipment available.
48. Decontamination from exposure.
49. Question and answer session.
50. Symptoms of blood-borne pathogen diseases.
51. State and OSHA rules.
52. Time of the meeting.
53. The exposure control plan.
54. Who gets HIV and AIDS.
55. Temperature that kills virus.
56. Give the coaches a list of athletes who are HIV-positive.
57. Redesign policy to restrict athletic competition by those with AIDS.
58. Disposal of contaminated equipment.
59. Preventing transmission.
60. Risks and benefits of an HBV vaccine.
61. Redesign policy to restrict athletic competition by those with HIV.
62. Identify coaches who have been exposed.

Problem 10

Opening Scene: An athlete has been referred to you by a physician after four months of unsuccessful rehabilitation. The athlete was an elite wrestler at the time of his knee injury. He is now six months post-surgical anterior cruciate repair. The physician's referral indicates athlete's injury was severs and return to competition is unlikely.

A. What is you initial assessment of this situation? (Choose only those actions that you have reason to believe are essential to the resolution of the problem at this time.)
   1. Ask athlete if he has pain currently.
   2. Ask athlete his goals for rehabilitation.
   3. Call emergency medical services.
   4. Ask when did it happen.
   5. Ask where was the pain initially.
   6. Introduce yourself.
   7. Ask did you hear or feel a pop, snap, crack, slip, or give at time of injury.
   8. Ask were you able to continue participating.
   9. Ask how soon after did it swell.
   10. Ask does it feel unstable.
   11. Ask what relieves the pain.
   12. Ask was your foot planted at the time of injury.
   13. Ask what treatment was given initially.
   14. Ask is there pain anywhere else.
   15. Ask how did it happen.

B. Given the information you have at this time, what would you do next to resolve this issue? (Choose only those actions that you have reason to believe are essential to the resolution of the problem at this time.)
   16. Check girth two inches above knee.
   17. Ask the athlete if he has been drinking.
   18. Check girth six inches above knee.
   19. Ask athlete if he has had any recent losses.
   20. Ask athlete about his eating habits.
   21. Check for swelling.
   22. Check for genu varum "bowlegged."
   23. Check for genu valgum "knock-knee."
   24. Check for deformity.
   25. Check for genu recurvatum "back knee."
   26. Check the scar.
   27. Check girth eight inches above knee.
   28. Check for pes planus and pes cavus.
   29. Check for tibia varus and valgus.
   30. Check for discoloration.
   31. Check for medial squinting of patella.
   32. Ask athlete about his sleeping habits.

C. Given the information you have at this time, what would you do next to resolve this issue? (Choose only those actions that you have reason to believe are essential to the resolution of the problem at this time.)
   33. Ask when was the last time you had thoughts of hurting yourself.
   34. Palpate the soft tissue.
   35. Palpate the medial meniscus.
   36. Palpate the popliteal space.
   37. Palpate the popliteal artery.
   38. Palpate the bony structures.
   39. Ask what kind of thoughts have you had lately.
   40. Palpate the joint line.
   41. Palpate the head of fibula.
   42. Palpate the lateral collateral ligament.
   43. Ask if he has had thoughts of hurting himself.
   44. Ask what has kept him from hurting himself.
   45. Palpate skin temperature.
   46. Palpate the medial joint line.
   47. Ask if he has any weapons.
   48. Ask if he has any plans to hurt himself today.

D. Given the information you have at this time, what would you do next to resolve this issue? (Choose only those actions that you have reason to believe are essential to the resolution of the problem at this time.)
   49. Determine athlete's insurance.
   50. Perform drawer test.
   51. Ask if he can avoid hurting himself in the next 24 hours.
   52. Perform Lachmans test.
   53. Perform apprehension test.
   54. Check abduction or external rotation.
   55. Give him the number to the crisis hotline.
   56. Ask for a phone number for a family member.
   57. Check range of motion.
   58. Check neurological function.
   59. Call athlete's family member.
   60. Begin massage therapy.
   61. Explain to athlete your goals for therapy.
   62. Place athlete in cold whirlpool.
   63. Apply electrical stimulation.
   64. Give a TENS unit for use at home.

Problem 11

Opening Scene: You have been hired for the first time to work with an adult men's lacrosse game, and are signaled onto the field.

A. What is your initial assessment of this situation? (Choose only those actions that you have reason to believe are essential to the resolution of the problem at this time.)
1. Remove athlete's helmet.
2. Grab your training kit.
3. Ask athlete what happened.
4. Roll the athlete while controlling the head and neck.
5. Determine if the athlete is conscious.
6. Determine if the athlete has a heartbeat.
7. Ask athlete if you can treat him.
8. Check the scene.
9. Remove face mask.
10. Determine if the airway is open.
11. Open airway using head tilt.
12. Remove athlete's helmet.
13. Determine if the athlete is breathing.
14. Carry athlete off the field.
15. Insert nasal cannula.
16. Stabilize the athlete's head and neck.
17. Remove athlete's mouth guard.

B. Given the information you have at this time, what would you do next to resolve this issue? (Choose only those actions that you have reason to believe are essential to the resolution of the problem at this time.)
18. Look for bleeding.
19. Straighten bones.
20. Call emergency medical technicians.
21. Check circulation at carotid.
22. Open airway.
23. Ask the athlete if you can treat him.
24. Watch athlete without treating him.
25. Check airway.
26. Elevate athlete's legs.

C. Given the information you have at this time, what would you do next to resolve this issue? (Choose only those actions that you have reason to believe are essential to the resolution of the problem at this time.)
27. Elevate both arms.
28. Apply direct pressure around the protruding bones.
29. Gently shake athlete calling his name.
30. Apply antiseptic to wound.
31. Check capillary refill.
32. Elevate the noninjured leg.
33. Give the athlete mouth-to-mouth resuscitation.
34. Apply sterile gauze to bones and wound.

35. Begin a secondary survey.
36. Apply direct pressure over fracture.
37. Splint the leg.
38. Elevate the athlete's head.

D. Given the information you have at this time, what would you do next to resolve this issue? (Choose only those actions that you have reason to believe are essential to the resolution of the problem at this time.)

39. Have athlete breathe into a paper bag.
40. Apply a blanket.
41. Re-splint the leg.
42. Elevate the splinted leg.
43. Insert an oral airway.
44. Begin intravenous saline.
45. Monitor airway, breathing, and circulation.
46. Check respiratory rate.
47. Allow emergency medical technicians to take over.
48. Take athlete's blood pressure.

Problem 12

Opening Scene: A rugby player who you treated initially, three days ago, with a thigh contusion has returned from the physician's office. The referral form indicates the athlete needs rehabilitation. He has decreased range of motion and strength, minimal pain, and some swelling.

A. What is your initial assessment of this situation? (Choose only those actions that you have reason to believe are essential to the resolution of the problem at this time.)

1. Check athlete's range of motion at the knee.
2. Determine strength.
3. Determine the diameter of the contusion.
4. Determine the girth of both thighs.
5. Determine the level of pain.
6. Determine range of motion at the hip.
7. Observe walking gait.
8. Determine the diameter of swelling.

B. Given the information you have at this time, what would you do next to resolve this issue? (Choose only those actions that you have reason to believe are essential to the resolution of the problem at this time.)

9. Apply muscle stimulation.
10. Apply biofeedback.
11. Apply ultrasound.
12. Apply laser.

13. Apply ice.
14. Massage.
15. Apply paraffin to leg.
16. Elevate body part.

C. Given the information you have at this time, what would you do next to resolve this issue? (Choose only those actions that you have reason to believe are essential to the resolution of the problem at this time.)

17. Four-way straight leg raises, no weights.
18. Quadriceps sets.
19. Squeezing a six-inch ball between knees.
20. Heel slides.
21. Apply ice after exercise.
22. Apply ultrasound.
23. Quadriceps stretching.

D. Given the information you have at this time, what would you do next to resolve this issue? (Choose only those actions that you have reason to believe are essential to the resolution of the problem at this time.)

24. Progressive resistive knee flexion exercises with weights.
25. Progressive resistive knee extension exercises with weights.
26. Return athlete to competition.
27. Four-way straight leg raises with weights.
28. Isokinetic exercises three days a week.
29. Plyometric depth jumping.
30. Quadriceps stretching.
31. Biking with seat elevated, two times per week.
32. Take athlete off crutches.
33. Upper body cycling.
34. Swimming.
35. Lateral step-ups.

E. Given the information you have at this time, what would you do next to resolve this issue? (Choose only those actions that you have reason to believe are essential to the resolution of the problem at this time.)

36. Squats.
37. Figure of eight drills.
38. Cutting drills.
39. Leg press exercises.
40. Running large circles.
41. Running small circles.
42. Jogging.

F. Given the information you have at this time, what would you do next to resolve this issue? (Choose only those actions that you have reason to believe are essential to the resolution of the problem at this time.)
   43. Tape thigh contusion area.
   44. PNF stretching.
   45. Leg press exercises.
   46. Pad the thigh.
   47. Block drills.
   48. Tackling drills.
   49. Slide board.
   50. Running sprints.
   51. Massage.
   52. Running a mile.
   53. Form running.
   53. Analgesic balm.
   55. Reaction drills.

G. Given the information you have at this time, how would you treat this athlete? (Choose only those actions that you have reason to believe are essential to the resolution of the problem at this time.)
   56. Leg press.
   57. Talk with athlete about need to pad thigh.
   58. Heat before practice.
   59. Pad the thigh.
   60. Talk with the coach about athlete's return.
   61. Ice after practice.

Problem 13

Opening Scene: A female gymnast that you cared for initially returns from Dr. Smith's office just having had a cast cut off her elbow. The physician's referral says the athlete was casted for a second-degree medial collateral ligament sprain. The physician indicates the athlete has limited flexion and pronation.

A. What is your initial assessment of this situation? (Choose only those actions that you have reason to believe are essential to the resolution of the problem at this time.)
   1. Ask how did it happen.
   2. Ask when did it happen.
   3. Ask where was the pain initially.
   4. Ask have you injured this before.
   5. Ask did you hear or feel a pop, snap, crack, slip, or give.
   6. Ask were you able to continue participating.
   7. Ask how soon after did it swell.
   8. Ask does it feel unstable.

9. Ask what relieves the pain.
10. Ask what treatment was given initially.
11. Ask who gave the treatment initially.
12. Ask the name of her physician.
13. Ask the athlete her goals.

B. Given the information you have at this time, what would you do next to resolve this issue? (Choose only those actions that you have reason to believe are essential to the resolution of the problem at this time.)
14. Look for dry skin.
15. Look for swelling.
16. Look for discoloration.
17. Look for deformity.
18. Look for valgus.
19. Look for scars.
20. Look for open sores.
21. Look for muscle atrophy bilaterally.
22. Look for varus.
23. Measure the forearm girth bilaterally.

C. Given the information you have at this time, what would you do next to resolve this issue? (Choose only those actions that you have reason to believe are essential to the resolution of the problem at this time.)
24. Check strength of medial collateral ligament.
25. Dress the pressure wound.
26. Palpate lateral collateral ligament.
27. Palpate medial epicondyle.
28. Check strength of lateral collateral ligament.
29. Check strength of annular ligament.
30. Check range of motion in flexion.
31. Check range of motion in pronation.
32. Check strength.
33. Check range of motion in radial deviation.
34. Check range of motion in ulnar deviation.
35. Check neurological sensation.
36. Palpate the medial collateral ligament.

D. Given the information you have at this time, what would you do next to resolve this issue? (Choose only those actions that you have reason to believe are essential to the resolution of the problem at this time.)
37. Ice the elbow.
38. Cold whirlpool while holding a heavy weight.
39. Have athlete perform PNF exercises for extension.
40. Have athlete perform PNF exercises for flexion.

41. Have athlete perform wall climb facing the wall.
42. Have athlete work with rope and pulley emphasizing flexion and extension of the elbow.
43. Begin an aerobic exercise program.
44. Have athlete perform isometrics at 0 degrees of extension.
45. Have athlete perform pendulum exercises.
46. Have athlete perform side wall climb.
47. Start a lower extremity strengthening program.
48. Begin passive stretching program.
49. Have athlete perform active-assistive wand stretching.
50. Have athlete perform isometrics at 120 degrees of flexion.

E. Given the information you have at this time, what would you do next to resolve this issue? (Choose only those actions that you have reason to believe are essential to the resolution of the problem at this time.)

51. Begin sport-specific activity of floor exercise.
52. Have athlete continue to perform rope and pulley.
53. Begin sport-specific activity of backward rolls.
54. Use the upper body extremity machine (UBE) for strengthening.
55. Have athlete perform empty can exercise with rubber tubing.
56. Continue aerobic exercise program.
57. Continue wall climbs.
58. Perform PNF flexion D1.
59. Begin isotonic strengthening with light dumbbells.
60. Begin sport-specific activity of forward rolls.
61. Perform PNF extension D2.
62. Continue lower extremity strengthening.
63. Perform PNF extension D1.
64. Perform PNF flexion D2.

F. Given the information you have at this time, what would you do next to resolve this issue? (Choose only those actions that you have reason to believe are essential to the resolution of the problem at this time.)

65. Begin weighted ball plyometrics.
66. Let the athlete begin dance portion of floor exercise.
67. Continue isotonic strengthening with heavier dumbbells.
68. Begin internal rotation isotonics.
69. Discontinue range of motion activities.
70. Begin overhead strengthening with light weights.
71. Perform PNF flexion D2.
72. Discontinue flexibility exercises.
73. Begin external rotation isotonics.
74. Begin jump training plyometrics.

75. Continue UBE strengthening.
76. Perform PNF extension D2.

G. Given the information you have at this time, what would you do next to resolve this issue? (Choose only those actions that you have reason to believe are essential to the resolution of the problem at this time.)
77. Restrict athlete to vault, beam, and floor exercise.
78. Have the athlete perform handstands.
79. Tape athlete's medial collateral ligament.
80. Allow athlete unrestricted return to activity.
81. Have the athlete ice after practice.
82. Have athlete see physician before return.
83. Restrict athlete to uneven bars.
84. Allow athlete to return to competition.

Problem 14

Opening Scene: You are a high school athletic trainer. A baseball player (outfielder) who you have evaluated and sent to the physician returns with a note. The note indicates the athlete has pain, full range of motion, and minimal decreased strength as a result of an acute first-degree rotator cuff strain. The physician desires control of pain and strengthening.

A. Given the information you have at this time, what would you do next to resolve this issue? (Choose only those actions that you have reason to believe are essential to the resolution of the problem at this time.)
1. Apply iontophoresis.
2. Apply heat to the area.
3. Ask athlete the location of the pain.
4. Begin active stretching.
5. Perform cross friction massage.
6. Apply laser.
7. Apply ice for 20 minutes.
8. Begin passive stretching.
9. Apply phonophoresis.
10. Have athlete perform wand exercises.
11. Apply ultrasound.
12. Apply electrical stimulation.
13. Have athlete perform on the upper body exerciser (UBE).
14. Give athlete ibuprofen.
15. Mobilize the shoulder.
16. Have athlete perform Codman pendulum exercises.
17. Place athlete in a sling.

B. Given the information you have at this time, what would you do next to resolve this issue? (Choose only those actions that you have reason to believe are essential to the resolution of the problem at this time.)

18. Continue icing the shoulder.
19. Have athlete perform empty can exercises with no resistance.
20. Have athlete perform isometric exercises.
21. Begin internal and external rotation exercises with light resistance.
22. Have athlete perform progressive resistive exercises for adduction.
23. Have the athlete perform with a body blade.
24. Have athlete perform progressive resistive exercises for internal rotation.
25. Have the athlete run on a treadmill.
26. Have athlete perform plyometric training.
27. Have athlete perform progressive resistive exercises for abduction.
28. Have athlete perform prone rows with light weights.
29. Have athlete stretch shoulder.
30. Have athlete perform progressive resistive exercises for external rotation with light resistance.

C. Given the information you have at this time, what would you do next to resolve this issue? (Choose only those actions that you have reason to believe are essential to the resolution of the problem at this time.)

31. Rest 10 minutes.
32. Have athlete throw 40 feet for 20 throws.
33. Apply analgesic pack.
34. Have athlete throw 60 feet for 20 throws.
35. Rest 10 minutes.
36. Have athlete perform flexion exercises with light weights.
37. Have athlete throw 60 feet for 20 throws.
38. Have athlete throw 40 feet for 20 throws.
39. Ice the shoulder.
40. Have athlete perform extension exercises with light weights.
41. Have athlete stretch shoulder.
42. Have athlete perform empty can exercises with light weights.

D. Given the information you have at this time, what would you do next to resolve this issue? (Choose only those actions that you have reason to believe are essential to the resolution of the problem at this time.)

43. Have athlete throw 90 feet for 20 throws.
44. Massage shoulder.
45. Have athlete throw 90 feet for 20 throws.
46. Have athlete rest 10 minutes.

47. Have athlete throw 60 feet for 20 throws.
48. Apply hydrocullator pack.
49. Have athlete throw 60 feet for 20 throws.
50. Have the athlete rest 10 minutes.
51. Have athlete perform pronation and supination exercises with weights.
52. Have athlete perform empty can exercises with progressive weights.

E. Given the information you have at this time, what would you do next to resolve this issue? (Choose only those actions that you have reason to believe are essential to the resolution of the problem at this time.)

53. Have athlete perform empty can exercises with progressive weights.
54. Have athlete throw 90 feet for 20 throws.
55. Ice the shoulder.
56. Have athlete throw 90 feet for 20 throws.
57. Have athlete stretch shoulder.
58. Have the athlete rest 10 minutes.
59. Have the athlete rest 10 minutes.
60. Have the athlete perform isometrics.

F. Given the information you have at this time, what would you do next to resolve this issue? (Choose only those actions that you have reason to believe are essential to the resolution of the problem at this time.)

61. Have athlete throw 125 feet for 20 throws.
62. Apply heat before throwing.
63. Have athlete throw 125 feet for 20 throws.
64. Have athlete perform empty can exercises with progressive weights.
65. Have the athlete rest 10 minutes.
66. Return athlete to full competition.
67. Have the athlete rest 10 minutes.
68. Ice the shoulder.
69. Have athlete stretch shoulder.

G. Given the information you have at this time, what would you do next to resolve this issue? (Choose only those actions that you have reason to believe are essential to the resolution of the problem at this time.)

70. Have athlete throw 150 feet for 20 throws.
71. Have athlete practice sliding.
72. Have athlete throw 150 feet for 20 throws.
73. Have athlete sprint 90 feet.
74. Have the athlete rest 10 minutes.

75. Return to active participation.
76. Have the athlete rest 10 minutes.
77. Ice the shoulder.
78. Have athlete take batting practice.

Problem 15

Opening Scene: You have been asked to design a program to increase the conditioning and strengthening of a wrestler on a high school team. The team wrestles three months of the year. He has just completed the season.

A. What is your initial assessment of this situation? (Choose only those actions that you have reason to believe are essential to the resolution of the problem at this time.)
   1. Skin fold test the wrestler.
   2. Determine the current upper body strength level of the wrestler.
   3. Determine the current lower body strength level of the wrestler.
   4. Determine flexibility of the wrestler.
   5. Determine current injuries of the wrestler.
   6. Determine aerobic fitness of the wrestler.
   7. Determine the balance of the wrestler.
   8. Determine anaerobic fitness of the wrestler.
   9. Begin intensive strengthening program.
   10. Determine the power of the wrestler.
   11. Let wrestler rest.
   12. Have wrestler do physical activities for fun.
   13. Determine heart rate of the wrestler.
   14. Have the wrestler take a physical.

B. Given the information you have at this time, what would you do next to resolve this issue? Choose only those actions that you have reason to believe are essential to the resolution of the problem at this time.
   15. Determine the nutritional intake of the wrestler.
   16. Determine water intake of the wrestler.
   17. Have the wrestler take an electrocardiogram.
   18. Skin fold test the wrestler.
   19. Determine the current upper body strength level of the wrestler.
   20. Determine the current lower body strength level of the wrestler.
   21. Determine flexibility of all wrestlers.
   22. Determine goniometic joint measurements.
   23. Determine aerobic fitness of the wrestler.
   24. Determine the balance of the wrestler.

25. Determine anaerobic fitness of the wrestler.
26. Determine heart rate of the wrestler.)
27. Determine the power of the wrestler.
28. Determine wrestlers previous training background.

C. Given the information you have at this time, what would you do next to resolve this issue? Choose only those actions that you have reason to believe are essential to the resolution of the problem at this time.

29. Have athlete perform leg extensions.
30. Have athlete perform leg curls.
31. Train at least four days per week.
32. Have athlete perform pull-ups.
33. Have athlete perform upright rows.
34. Actively rest.
35. Have athlete perform snatches.
36. Have athlete perform deadlifts.
37. Train at least three days per week.
38. Have athlete perform stiff-leg deadlift.
39. Have athlete perform push-ups.
40. Have athlete perform weighted step-ups.
41. Have athlete perform lunges.
42. Have athlete perform triceps pushdowns.
43. Have athlete perform front squats.
44. Have athlete perform back squats.
45. Have athlete perform hip sled strengthening.
46. Have athlete perform wrist extension strengthening.
47. Have athlete perform wrist flexion strengthening.
48. Have athlete perform incline dumbbell bench presses.
49. Have athlete perform inline dumbbell fly.
50. Have athlete perform calf raises.
51. Have athlete perform hammer curl.
52. Have athlete perform seated rows.
53. Have athlete perform biceps curls.
54. Have athlete perform lat pull downs.
55. Have athlete perform bent-over row.
56. Have athlete perform crunches.
57. Have athlete perform bent-knee sit-up.
58. Have athlete perform shoulder press.
59. Have athlete run a mile every other day.
60. Have athlete run sprints every other day.
61. Have athlete perform power cleans.

D. Given the information you have at this time, and knowing this is just prior to pre-season what would you do next to resolve this issue? Choose only those actions that you have reason to believe are essential to the resolution of the problem at this time.
   62. Have the athlete perform sport specific weight training.
   63. Have the athlete perform wrestling drills.
   64. Have athlete continue weight training.
   65. Have the athlete participate in recreational sports other than wrestling.
   66. Have athlete run a mile every other day.
   67. Have athlete run sprints every other day.
   68. Have the athlete actively rest.

E. Given the information you have at this time, and know that it is now pre-season what would you do next to resolve this issue? (Choose only those actions that you have reason to believe are essential to the resolution of the problem at this time.)
   69. Increase agility.
   70. Increase power.
   71. Increase strength.
   72. Do a circuit training.
   73. Lift weights for maintenance.
   74. Lift three to four times per week.
   75. Perform anaerobic running.
   76. Improve balance.
   77. Perform aerobic workout.
   78. Have athlete run a mile every other day.
   79. Work on wrestling techniques.

Problem 16

Opening Scene: A physician has sent you a golfer who wants to begin functional sport-specific activity. The athlete had a second degree quadratus lumborum strain.

A. What is your initial assessment of this situation? (Choose only those actions that you have reason to believe are essential to the resolution of the problem at this time.)
   1. Ask if he has any shooting pains.
   2. Ask athlete if he has pain with motion.
   3. Ask if he was able to continue playing.
   4. Check his breathing rate.
   5. Ask how he hurt himself.
   6. Ask what makes him comfortable.
   7. Ask what he has been doing to treat his back.

8. Ask if he has injured his back before.
9. Check is pulse rate.
10. Determine course he was playing at the time of injury.
11. Ask when did injury occur.
12. Ask his golf handicap.

B. Given the information you have at this time, what would you do next to resolve this issue? (Choose only those actions that you have reason to believe are essential to the resolution of the problem at this time.)
13. Check trunk flexion.
14. Check his ability to touch his toes.
15. Check right lateral bending from side lying.
16. Check trunk extension prone.
17. Check hip abduction.
18. Check hip adduction.
19. Check rotation left.
20. Check rotation right.
21. Check hip flexion.
22. Check hip extension.
23. Check inguinal ligament.
24. Check lateral bending left.
25. Check lateral bending right.
26. Check right lateral bending from side lying.
27. Check trunk extension standing.

C. Given the information you have at this time, what would you do next to resolve this issue? (Choose only those actions that you have reason to believe are essential to the resolution of the problem at this time.)
28. Test flexibility of hip flexors.
29. Have athlete perform straight leg raising test.
30. Test flexibility of Achilles tendon.
31. Perform Hoover test for malingering.
32. Test Gaensien's sign.
33. Perform pelvic rock compression test.
34. Patrick or Fabere test.
35. Check leg length.
36. Test flexibility of quadratus lumborum.
37. Test stretching of femoral nerve.
38. Perform the Milgram test.
39. Observe walking gait.
40. Have athlete perform Ober test.

D. Given the information you have at this time, what would you recommend to this athlete to resolve this issue? (Choose only those actions that you have reason to believe are essential to the resolution of the problem at this time.)

41. Stretch upper extremity muscles.
42. Touches toes with feet shoulder width apart.
43. Rotate left from golf stance.
44. Stretch wrists into extension.
45. Stretch lateral trunk muscles bilaterally.
46. Stretch the anterior muscles of the tibia.
47. Stretch trunk rotator muscles bilaterally.
48. Rotate right from golf stance.

E. Given the information you have at this time, what would you do next to resolve this issue? Choose only those actions that you have reason to believe are essential to the resolution of the problem at this time.

49. Chipping for 10 minutes.
50. Throwing a club 10 times.
51. Driver swings for three minutes.
52. Pick up golf bag and carry 20 yards.
53. Pitching wedge swings for three minutes.
54. Iron swings for three minutes.
55. Putting for 10 minutes.
56. Deep grass shots for three minutes.

F. Given the information you have at this time, what would you recommend to prevent re-injury? Choose only those actions that you have reason to believe are essential to the resolution of the problem at this time.

57. Golf stretches.
58. Bent-over rows.
59. Back lying with hip-hiking exercise.
60. Interval training.
61. Standing hip-hiking exercise.
62. Hyperextension exercises.
63. Back lying with hip-hiking exercise against manual resistance.
64. Lat pull downs.
65. None.
66. Crunches.
67. Walking instead of using a cart.

Problem 17

Opening Scene: You are covering an ice hockey game. Between periods, in the locker room, a player complains that he's not feeling well. You have a headache.

A. What is your initial assessment of this situation? Choose only those actions that you have reason to believe are essential to the resolution of the problem at this time.

1. Ask athlete if he hit his head.
2. He says nothing he can remember, but a couple of other guys also feel the same way.
3. Ask where was the pain initially.
4. Ask if he knew who hit him.
5. Ask how does he feel.
6. Were you able to continue participating.
7. Check airway.
8. Ask why he has not come in before.
9. Ask what relieves the pain.
10. Ask what treatment was given initially
11. Ask how he has headaches.
12. Ask if he injured this before.
13. Ask if he takes medication.
14. Ask what did you eat today.
15. Ask how soon after did it swell.
16. Check for bleeding.
17. Ask "When did it happen?"
18. Look, listen and feel for breathing.
19. Survey the scene.
20. Check pulse rate.
21. Ask if anyone else has a headache or feels dizzy.
22. Ask if the athlete is nauseous.
23. Check level of consciousness.
24. Ask if anyone on the team has been sick lately.

B. Given the information you have at this time, what would you do next to resolve this issue? Choose only those actions that you have reason to believe are essential to the resolution of the problem at this time.

25. Give athlete aspirin.
26. Check for deformity, depression.
27. Determine what was eaten by the rest of the team.
28. Look for leakage of cerebrospinal fluid.
29. Check for aphasia.
30. Check breathing pattern and rates.
31. Check for nystagmus.
32. Check for swelling.
33. Call emergency medical system for help.
34. Check for discoloration.
35. Check for battle sign.
36. Check mouth for foreign object.
37. Check pupillary reflex.

C. Given the information you have at this time, what would you do next to resolve this issue? Choose only those actions that you have reason to believe are essential to the resolution of the problem at this time.
   38. Palpate the skull.
   39. Palpate the jaw.
   40. Palpate the facial bones.
   41. Take team outside.
   42. Perform a secondary survey.
   43. Check athlete's blood pressure.
   44. Take the team out of the locker room into hallway.
   45. Take athlete's temperature.

D. Given the information you have at this time, what would you do next to resolve this issue? (Choose only those actions that you have reason to believe are essential to the resolution of the problem at this time.)
   46. Have athlete drink lots of water.
   47. Have athlete drink a glass of orange juice.
   48. Cool athlete with towels.
   49. Ask the manager to evacuate the arena.
   50. Stop the game.
   51. Sit the athlete out a period.
   52. Return to the bench for the second period.
   53. Give the athlete antacids.
   54. Give athlete syrup of ipecac.
   55. Send athlete to hospital.
   56. Send whole team to hospital.

E. Given the information you have at this time, what is the cause of the athletes' illness? (Choose only those actions that you have reason to believe are essential to the resolution of the problem at this time.)
   57. Ulcer.
   58. Seizure.
   59. Carbon monoxide poisoning.
   60. Heat exhaustion.
   61. Food poisoning.
   62. Head injury.
   63. Influenza.
   64. Gastroenteritis.

Problem 18

Opening Scene: You're covering a 20-team middle-school cross-country invitational. You are radioed that there's an athlete injured on the field.

A. What is your initial assessment of this situation? (Choose only those actions that you have reason to believe are essential to the resolution of the problem at this time.)

1. Run to the athlete.
2. Ask what the injury might be.
3. Tell people you are unable to leave your area.
4. Send a student athletic trainer to cover your area of the course.
5. Determine where the injured athlete is on the course.
6. Determine the uniform color of the last runner.
7. Determine the school of the athlete that is injured.
8. Call for the golf cart to come and get you.
9. Ask the color of the team jersey.
10. Grab your training kit.

B. Given the information you have at this time, what would you do next to resolve this issue? (Choose only those actions that you have reason to believe are essential to the resolution of the problem at this time.)

11. Determine the status of the race.
12. Call for an ambulance.
13. Radio to determine where the athlete is located.
14. Check the position of the athlete.
15. Radio course officials and let them know you are working hard.
16. Walk the last half of the course.
17. Make sure you have your sunglasses.
18. Have all course officials determine location of any down athletes.
19. Check to be sure the scene is safe.
20. Ask the coach if she is missing an athlete.
21. Ask for medical identification card.
22. Ask the coach if anyone is injured.
23. Ask coach the nature of athlete's injury.
24. Make sure you have your identification.
25. Determine the location of athletes' parents.
26. Go back to your spot on the course.

C. Given the information you have at this time, what would you do next to resolve this issue? (Choose only those actions that you have reason to believe are essential to the resolution of the problem at this time.)

27. Ask the athlete if you can help her (she is alert but refuses to talk with you.)
28. Call for an ambulance.
29. Go to the athlete.
30. Check airway.
31. Ask the father if you can help.
32. Check breathing.
33. Ask the parent the original location of the athlete.
34. Ask the parents to sign a waiver declining care.
35. Ask the mother if you can help.

36. Ask teammates what happened.
37. Leave the area.

D. Given the information you have at this time, what would you do next to resolve this issue? Choose only those actions that you have reason to believe are essential to the resolution of the problem at this time.
38. Ask parents if this injury as happened before.
39. Leave scene.
40. Give care to emergency medical technicians.
41. Get a witness.
42. Ask the parents to sign a waiver declining care.
43. Question the emergency medical technicians.
44. Determine the location of the coach.
45. Get the name and address of the witness.
46. Go to the finish line.
47. Apologize to the family.

E. Given the information you have at this time, what would you do next to resolve this issue? Choose only those actions that you have reason to believe are essential to the resolution of the problem at this time.
48. Ask the coach the name of the girl.
49. Ask the coach if she knows the condition of the athlete.
50. Return to your spot on the course.
51. Call your athletic director.
52. Ask for the athlete's address.
53. Eat a power food bar.
54. Ask for the athlete's phone number.
55. Worry that you'll be sued.
56. Document the situation.
57. Talk to another person to debrief about the incident.
58. Call the family at home.
59. Determine the hospital of choice.

F. You are called to the athletic directors office the next day. Given the information you have at this time, what would you do next to resolve this issue? Choose only those actions that you have reason to believe are essential to the resolution of the problem at this time.
60. Provide documentation of the situation.
61. Indicate athlete was moved.
62. Indicate you're unsure of the diagnosis.
63. Give the name of the school
64. Indicate athlete's name.
65. Call the local hospitals.
66. Ask your team physician to call the local hospitals.

G. The athletic director asks you to prepare an emergency plan to ensure prompt care before the next race in seven days. Given the information you have at this time, what would you do next to resolve this issue?
   67. Present plan to athletic director.
   68. Get a map of the course.
   69. Have a radio system to track race.
   70. Send letter to all attending schools.
   71. Determine the number of staff members
   72. Get some keys.
   73. Place people on the map equal distance.
   74. Determine field conditions.
   75. Make sure all athletic training staff have radios.
   76. Determine level of care necessary.
   77. Determine how to remove an athlete from the course.
   78. Determine who will do debriefing.
   79. Determine who does what in an injury.
   80. Determine obstacles.
   81. Get the phone numbers of the various schools involved.
   82. Practice the plan.
   83. Purchase bolt cutters.
   84. Determine who will give counseling.
   85. Make sure all staff have identifiable gear.
   86. Determine the site of triage.
   87. Determine supplies necessary.
   88. Make sure there is water for participants.
   89. Determine the access entry area for an ambulance.
   90. Determine the number of participants.
   91. Repair the tire on the golf cart.
   92. Make sure you have back-up batteries.
   93. Go over who covers what areas on map.

Problem 19

Opening Scene: You're at a baseball game, and the catcher misses a foul fly ball. The umpire summons you onto the field.

A. What is your initial response to this situation? Choose only those actions that you have reason to believe are essential to the resolution of the case at this time.
   1. Pick up the catcher's face mask.
   2. Ask athlete if pain any place other than already noted.
   3. Call athlete's parents.
   4. Ask athlete to roll onto his back.
   5. Have the athlete tilt his head back.
   6. Ask athlete to explain what happened.

7. Open athlete's airway.
8. Begin giving mouth-to-mouth breathing.
9. Begin CPR.
10. Determine athlete's level of consciousness.
11. Ask the athlete about the pain.
12. Visually examine the position of the catcher.

B. Given the previous information how would you proceed at this time. (Choose only those action that you have reason to believe are essential to the resolution of the case at this time)
13. Check the athlete's teeth.
14. Check athletes body temperature.
15. Determine skin color.
16. Ask about previous injuries.
17. Apply ice.
18. Remove the airway obstruction.

C. What is your initial treatment of this situation? Choose only those action that you have reason to believe are essential to the resolution of the case at this time.
19. Give athlete a couple of aspirins,
20. Apply ice.
21. Put the athlete back into the game.
22. Apply sterile gauze and direct pressure.
23. Clean the athlete's uniform.
24. Palpate facial bones.
25. Continue mouth-to-mouth breathing.
26. Look at the cut.
27. Call for an ambulance.
28. Hold the athlete's head and neck.

D. What is your additional assessment, given the previous information. Choose only those actions that you have reason to believe are essential to the resolution of the case at this time.
29. Put the athlete back in the game.
30. Check athlete's pupils.
31. Call for an ambulance.
32. Backboard the athlete.
33. Ask the coach how soon he needs the athlete.
34. Ask the athlete if they have a ride home
35. Apply a soft collar.
36. Ask the athlete the score
37. Check for tinnitus.
38. Ask if the athlete is nauseous.
39. Check athlete's balance.

40. Have athlete take a few warm-up tosses and swing a bat.

E. What is your overnight recommendation for this athlete and his parents? Choose only those actions that you have reason to believe are essential to the resolution of the case at this time.
   41. Give aspirin every two hours.
   42. Awaken every two hours.
   43. Watch for vomiting.
   44. Apply ice all night.
   45. Send to the emergency room if condition gets worse.
   46. Athlete should be hospitalized over night.
   47. Check blood pressure every two hours.
   48. Check athlete's temperature.
   49. Keep athlete walking around all night.
   50. Have athlete sleep with head elevated.
   51. Check athletes hearing every two hours.
   52. Apply topical antibiotic ointment.
   53. Watch athlete for uncharacteristic behavioral changes.
   54. Seek the assistance of a physician.

Problem 20

Opening scene: A high school wrestler reports to you that he has several round circles of a rash all over his head, neck, and face.

A. Given the information you have at this time, what would you do next to resolve this issue? Choose only those actions that you have reason to believe are essential to the resolution of the problem at this time.
   1. Put on goggles and a face mask.
   2. Ask how long athlete has had the rash.
   3. Apply antiseptic to rash.
   4. Put on latex gloves.
   5. Ask if athlete knows where he got it.
   6. Contact the coach and determine how often mats are cleaned.
   7. Take athlete's temperature.
   8. Wash your hands.
   9. Disinfect area where evaluation of athlete took place. (not necessary at this time)
   10. Determine age of athlete's brother.
   11. Examine the rash.

B. Given the information you have at this time, what would you do next to resolve this issue? Choose only those actions that you have reason to believe are essential to the resolution of the problem at this time.
   12. Cover the rash.
   13. Apply antifungal medication.

14. Refer athlete to physician.
15. Send athlete home.
16. Disinfect the entire training room.

C. The physician calls to say the athlete has tinea capitis. Given the information you have at this time, what would you do next to resolve this issue? Choose only those actions that you have reason to believe are essential to the resolution of the problem at this time.

17. No further action is necessary.
18. Have someone disinfect athlete's locker.
19. Have athletes stop using others equipment.
20. Determine all athletes that wrestler competed against.
21. Send all wrestlers home.
22. Have mats disinfected with bleach.
23. Check all athletes' immunization records.
24. Report case to communicable disease office at county health department.
25. Close the school.
26. Contact all schools the wrestling team competed against.
27. Contact school medical staff.
28. Issue an educational sheet on spread of disease.
29. Send home and educational sheet to parents about signs.
30. Send home and exclude all students from school who have not been immunized.
31. Fumigate school.
32. Contact local newspaper.
33. Remind all students to cover their mouths.
34. Quickly examine all wrestlers for possible signs.
35. Make sure athletes use cups rather than water bottles.

D. The original wrestler calls to say he is coming in. Given the information you have at this time, what would you do next to resolve this issue? Choose only those actions that you have reason to believe are essential to the resolution of the case at this time.

36. Athlete can return once the school nurse gives him the ok.
37. Athlete can return once he gets immunized.
38. Athlete can return once as soon as the coach needs him.
39. Encourage athlete to use medication.
40. Educate athlete on sanitary procedures.
41. Return athlete to competition without any issue.
42. Allow athlete to return with physician's permission.

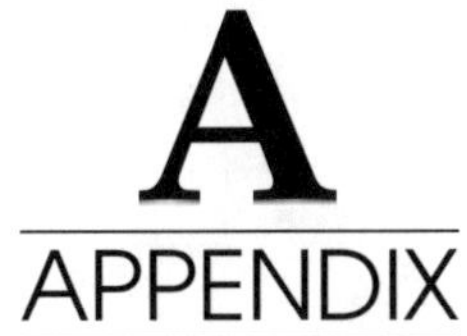

APPENDIX

Answer Key for the Written Examination Study Questions

References and page numbers refer to bibliography starting on page 202.

	Answer	Reference	Page Number
Prevention			
1.	b	24	142
2.	b	24	142
3.	d	24	152
4.	c	67	60
5.	c	34	36
6.	c	34	36
7.	b	34	36
8.	c	34	65
9.	e	34	64
10.	c	34	35
11.	c	34	35
12.	e	34	65
13.	b	34	43-44
14.	e	89	267
15.	b	89	264
16.	a	26	248
17.	e	26	256
18.	b	26	256
19.	b	26	258
20.	b	23	69
21.	e	26	259
22.	b	23	38
23.	a	26	271
24.	e	88	664
25.	a	86	640
26.	c	80	79
27.	e	34	23
28.	e	84	28
29.	e	31	34
30.	c	31	2
31.	b	31	12
32.	d	31	16
33.	e	31	21
34.	c	31	23
35.	e	13	161
36.	d	31	52
37.	e	13	153-154
38.	b	2	159
39.	e	14	560
40.	a	31	57
41.	b	31	58
42.	a	89	211
43.	d	2	142
44.	b	2	130
45.	d	31	78
46.	e	14	384-385
47.	a	29	232
48.	e	31	87
49.	e	47	101
50.	a	23	24
51.	c	31	97

	Answer	Reference	Page Number
52.	b	31	98
53.	a	23	298
54.	e	14	244
55.	e	31	103
56.	e	14	247
57.	b	31	113
58.	b	89	748
59.	c	75	43
60.	c	31	125
61.	e	31	125
62.	e	29	238
63.	e	14	255
64.	b	31	143
65.	b	31	152
66.	c	23	205
67.	d	14	254
68.	a	86	130
69.	a	31	264
70.	a	89	988
71.	c	23	262
72.	d	23	139
73.	e	23	25
74.	d	23	105
75.	e	31	205
76.	b	89	190
77.	b	31	207
78.	c	89	211
79.	d	31	209
80.	d	75	211
81.	d	14	254
82.	b	88	582-585
83.	d	31	213
84.	c	75	230
85.	c	23	104
86.	b	13	24
87.	d	23	137
88.	c	13	23
89.	c	31	241
90.	d	13	45
91.	d	14	50
92.	b	23	111

Passing point total: 65

Recognition, Evaluation, and Assessment

	Answer	Reference	Page Number
93.	a	23	448
94.	c	9	366
95.	d	38	4
96.	a	38	13-15
97.	b	38	21
98.	c	38	39
99.	d	8	111
100.	a	38	46
101.	b	13	525
102.	a	80	390
103.	c	8	110
104.	a	80	82
105.	e	38	64
106.	b	80	425
107.	c	26	293
108.	e	75	38
109.	e	16	216
110.	a	75	295-296
111.	a	38	85
112.	a	38	93
113.	b	38	96
114.	e	38	104
115.	d	38	105
116.	b	2	448
117.	b	75	300
118.	c	38	127
119.	e	38	129
120.	d	38	131
121.	c	38	132-133
122.	e	23	302-303
123.	b	38	142-143
124.	e	21	75
125.	c	38	160-161
126.	d	38	181
127.	c	21	356
128.	a	38	187
129.	c	8	111
130.	e	26	317
131.	d	38	214
132.	c	26	258
133.	a	38	220
134.	c	13	733
135.	e	80	36
136.	d	38	227-228
137.	c	13	115
138.	b	80	282
139.	a	13	540-541
140.	c	38	243
141.	d	80	430
142.	b	38	252-253
143.	e	38	260
144.	c	38	262

	Answer	Reference	Page Number
145.	a	38	265
146.	e	24	157
147.	c	80	61
148.	d	24	305
149.	a	8	641
150.	b	8	642
151.	d	8	679
152.	d	8	612
153.	a	8	656
154.	c	8	654
155.	d	2	298
156.	a	8	635
157.	e	8	658
158.	e	8	658
159.	a	8	528
160.	b	8	661
161.	e	8	642
162.	a	8	663
163.	a	13	117
164.	b	13	117
165.	c	8	657
166.	b	8	635
167.	e	9	341-342
168.	a	8	111
169.	b	8	660
170.	b	8	75
171.	a	8	642
172.	a	8	64
173.	d	8	180
174.	e	8	665
175.	d	8	665
176.	d	8	666
177.	a	8	666
178.	e	8	653
179.	b	8	654
180.	e	8	604
181.	e	8	63
182.	b	75	128
183.	b	8	651-652
184.	a	8	59
185.	a	75	128
186.	d	2	445
187.	a	2	446
188.	d	2	448
189.	b	2	480
190.	a	2	480
191.	b	2	556
192.	d	2	556
193.	a	8	37
194.	e	2	903
195.	b	80	336
196.	c	2	860
197.	b	2	570
198.	b	2	450
199.	e	2	90
200.	a	2	90
201.	a	2	93
202.	b	8	111-112
203.	b	8	42
204.	b	8	510
205.	b	2	501-502
206.	d	75	149
207.	e	75	128
208.	e	2	501
209.	c	8	528
210.	d	8	530
211.	e	8	530
212.	d	8	526
213.	a	8	522
214.	e	13	115
215.	e	8	506
216.	b	8	503
217.	a	8	503-504
218.	c	8	503
219.	a	8	519-520
220.	a	8	520
221.	c	8	653
222.	b	8	527
223.	a	8	238
224.	b	8	392
225.	d	8	409
226.	e	8	409
227.	b	8	383
228.	d	8	440-441

Passing point total: 95

Immediate Care

	Answer	Reference	Page Number
229.	a	23	69
230.	b	23	69
231.	e	23	68
232.	e	23	71
233.	c	23	71
234.	c	23	71
235.	d	23	745
236.	b	23	74
237.	d	23	79

	Answer	Reference	Page Number
238.	a	23	109
239.	e	23	121
240.	c	23	147
241.	e	23	377
242.	d	23	150
243.	a	23	157
244.	e	23	158
245.	b	23	186
246.	d	23	205
247.	a	23	209
248.	d	23	213
249.	b	23	215
250.	c	23	224
251.	a	23	604
252.	e	23	271
253.	e	23	286
254.	c	47	43
255.	b	47	45
256.	e	23	375
257.	b	23	380
258.	d	23	381
259.	a	23	605
260.	d	23	382-384
261.	b	23	396
262.	b	23	397
263.	b	23	408
264.	c	47	105
265.	b	23	311
266.	a	23	444
267.	b	23	299
268.	b	23	449
269.	c	13	411
270.	c	23	72
271.	d	23	547
272.	b	23	565
273.	a	23	651
274.	a	23	658
275.	a	8	529
276.	b	8	529
277.	e	8	528
278.	b	13	414
279.	e	8	520-521
280.	a	8	524
281.	e	8	524
282.	c	8	526
283.	a	8	383
284.	e	86	638
285.	e	13	429
286.	b	80	474
287.	d	80	367-368
288.	a	23	570
289.	a	13	279
290.	a	13	304
291.	c	13	279
292.	e	8	524
293.	c	8	526
294.	d	9	319
295.	d	80	121
296.	c	37	89
297.	a	37	36
298.	a	37	36
299.	a	37	37
300.	e	37	68
301.	d	37	95
302.	c	37	192
303.	d	37	192
304.	b	37	247
305.	a	28	28
306.	e	23	277
307.	b	23	277
308.	c	23	272
309.	e	2	448
310.	e	33	13-17
311.	d	23	454
312.	c	2	141
313.	a	2	221
314.	e	2	220
315.	c	2	219-220
316.	c	2	220
317.	c	2	208-209
318.	d	23	453
319.	a	23	366-367
320.	a	23	165-166
321.	c	23	168
322.	a	91	30-38
323.	d	23	118
324.	c	23	398-399
325.	b	23	395
326.	e	13	429
327.	c	23	453-454
328.	a	23	278
329.	d	23	278
330.	c	13	591
331.	a	13	587
332.	a	23	348-349
333.	a	23	651

	Answer	Reference	Page Number
334.	b	13	554
335.	a	23	576
336.	a	86	616
337.	c	86	618
338.	c	80	369
339.	d	71	257
340.	d	9	558
341.	a	9	68
342.	b	9	92
343.	e	89	270
344.	b	89	270
345.	e	71	257-263
346.	c	2	588
347.	e	2	588
348.	c	23	659
349.	c	2	215
350.	b	13	856
351.	c	69	21
352.	b	69	40
353.	a	23	57
354.	a	69	187
355.	d	69	196
356.	e	69	332

Passing point total: 90

Treatment, Rehabilitation, and Reconditioning

	Answer	Reference	Page Number
357.	d	28	27
358.	a	69	3
359.	e	72	390
360.	c	69	5
361.	e	69	7
362.	c	69	8
363.	d	69	14
364.	c	69	14
365.	a	69	14
366.	c	69	16
367.	b	69	16
368.	a	69	16
369.	c	69	16
370.	b	8	178
371.	c	69	20
372.	c	69	20
373.	d	72	413
374.	e	69	22
375.	a	13	733
376.	b	89	564
377.	b	72	513
378.	a	69	25
379.	c	37	49
380.	c	69	25
381.	d	69	25
382.	c	69	26
383.	c	69	26
384.	a	69	34
385.	e	69	34
386.	e	69	35
387.	c	69	35
388.	b	69	35
389.	c	69	35
390.	a	69	36
391.	a	72	514
392.	c	69	44
393.	c	29	64
394.	a	29	64
395.	a	31	212
396.	d	8	77
397.	b	29	86
398.	d	29	165
399.	e	28	29
400.	a	75	130
401.	a	75	147
402.	a	75	208
403.	a	35	88
404.	b	35	88
405.	a	69	98
406.	a	69	99
407.	a	69	100
408.	c	37	41
409.	c	89	247
410.	d	69	186
411.	c	72	388
412.	d	75	267
413.	a	72	330
414.	d	69	198
415.	e	85	98
416.	c	69	200
417.	d	75	128-130
418.	e	2	448
419.	c	69	203
420.	c	2	887
421.	e	2	480
422.	d	8	259
423.	a	69	270
424.	a	72	185
425.	c	72	316

	Answer	Reference	Page Number
426.	b	72	281
427.	d	69	269
428.	c	72	166
429.	b	69	279
430.	a	9	319
431.	a	69	345
432.	c	69	345
433.	c	85	236
434.	c	69	298
435.	a	69	307
436.	a	2	446
437.	d	69	313
438.	e	69	315
439.	c	75	158
440.	d	69	325
441.	b	37	57
442.	c	69	327
443.	e	69	127
444.	a	69	129
445.	c	69	124
446.	d	69	87
447.	a	69	85
448.	e	69	20
449.	b	69	20
450.	a	69	324-325
451.	d	69	324-325
452.	c	5	59
453.	a	5	58
454.	c	5	89-92
455.	c	69	235
456.	e	67	121
457.	a	69	277
458.	c	24	112
459.	d	24	112
460.	b	24	112
461.	a	24	113
462.	c	24	113
463.	c	4	8
464.	d	4	6-7
465.	a	85	214
466.	a	24	115
467.	e	24	115-116
468.	e	24	118
469.	a	24	119
470.	d	24	120
471.	d	24	120
472.	b	24	121
473.	c	24	123
474.	c	24	126
475.	e	24	126
476.	a	24	130
477.	a	24	130
478.	c	24	130
479.	d	24	139
480.	d	24	140
481.	d	24	254
482.	b	24	309
483.	d	84	43
484.	b	84	76-77
485.	e	84	79
486.	e	84	16
487.	b	84	17
488.	d	84	84

Passing point total: 92

Organization and Administration

	Answer	Reference	Page Number
489.	c	76	161
490.	a	76	161
491.	c	76	117
492.	d	76	161
493.	c	76	161
494.	b	13	408
495.	b	76	162
496.	b	76	162
497.	d	76	162
498.	d	76	163
499.	c	76	123
500.	a	76	163
501.	a	76	163
502.	e	76	164-174
503.	a	76	164
504.	a	76	137
505.	a	76	166
506.	e	76	147
507.	b	76	168-169
508.	c	76	169
509.	c	76	169-170
510.	b	76	170-171
511.	a	76	170-171
512.	e	76	173
513.	a	76	173
514.	c	76	174
515.	a	76	174
516.	d	76	174
517.	d	76	174
518.	a	76	178

	Answer	Reference	Page Number
519.	b	76	178
520.	a	76	179
521.	e	76	179
522.	b	76	179
523.	c	76	29-30
524.	b	76	32-33
525.	a	76	5
526.	b	76	14
527.	e	76	32
528.	c	75	158
529.	c	75	158
530.	d	75	157
531.	c	76	202
532.	d	76	67
533.	a	75	221
534.	e	76	202
535.	d	75	163
536.	d	73	17
537.	b	73	23
538.	a	73	24-25
539.	d	73	42
540.	e	73	42
541.	d	73	147
542.	a	75	15-16
543.	c	76	195
544.	a	75	137
545.	a	76	108
546.	c	76	16
547.	e	76	27
548.	a	76	37

Passing point total: 42

Professional Development

	Answer	Reference	Page Number
549.	e	76	68-69
550.	b	51	5
551.	d	51	5
552.	b	51	5
553.	e	51	5
554.	e	51	5
555.	d	51	5
556.	b	51	5
557.	c	59	1
558.	a	59	3
559.	b	59	3
560.	c	59	2
561.	a	73	217
562.	a	59	3
563.	d	59	3
564.	c	59	3
565.	e	59	1
566.	e	59	2
567.	e	59	2
568.	c	59	2
569.	a	59	2
570.	e	59	4
571.	c	59	4
572.	b	59	4
573.	b	76	178
574.	e	76	226
575.	d	76	186-189
576.	e	73	222
577.	a	76	98-99
578.	b	61	1
579.	b	52	3
580.	b	73	222
581.	d	73	214-218
582.	c	76	196
583.	d	13	31
584.	b	76	234
585.	b	13	64
586.	b	13	64
587.	b	13	408
588.	b	13	408
589.	a	13	439
590.	d	13	440
591.	c	62	1
592.	d	22	139
593.	a	22	131
594.	e	22	141
595.	e	76	223-225
596.	a	33	10
597.	e	76	279
598.	a	73	216
599.	c	34	57
600.	e	76	77

Passing point total: 36

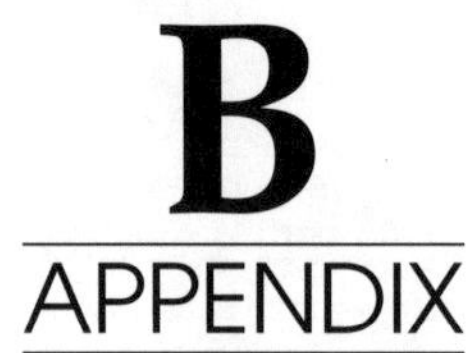

APPENDIX

Answers to the Study Questions for the Practical Test

The following checklist will help you be sure that you thoroughly cover all necessary points when demonstrating a response to the question on the practical section of the exam. To use this checklist, have a partner read and show you the questions, which appear in chapter 7.

As you demonstrate the proper response, have your partner indicate, by placing a check mark in the appropriate box, where you made the appropriate response that count for points on the exam. Remember you will not receive points for explaining anything—you must demonstrate. You have only one opportunity to perform the task correctly. At the end of the response section it says "completes this task in X minutes or less." The response does not have a yes/no response as by not completing the task will result in the loss of points. At the end of each question is the passing-point total. Have your partner add together all yes answers and compare them to the passing-point total. The point totals are 70% of points possible for that question.

1. Application of Skin Closures.

Applies latex gloves	❑ Yes	❑ No
Skin surface is dry before application	❑ Yes	❑ No
Peels closures off in a diagonal direction	❑ Yes	❑ No
Applies tincture of benzoin on both sides of wound	❑ Yes	❑ No
Applies closures from the same side to the other	❑ Yes	❑ No
Applies closures pulling skin together	❑ Yes	❑ No

Applies closures starting at the center of the wound working outward ❑ Yes ❑ No

Applies closures one eighth of an inch apart ❑ Yes ❑ No

Completes task in three minutes or less

Passing-point total: 6

Reference: 91, pp. 25-27

2. Assessing Breath Sounds.

Athlete is placed in a seated supine or prone position ❑ Yes ❑ No

Listens to breath at midclavicular sites ❑ Yes ❑ No

Listens to breath sounds at midaxillary sites ❑ Yes ❑ No

Listens to breath sounds at nipple level site ❑ Yes ❑ No

Listens to breath sounds at lower rib site ❑ Yes ❑ No

Listens to equal breath sounds bilaterally (midclavicular to midclavicular, and midaxillary to midaxillary) ❑ Yes ❑ No

Completes task in five minutes or less

Passing-point total: 4

Reference: 16, pp. 143-144

3. Use of a Sling Psychrometer.

Dampens the wet bulb ❑ Yes ❑ No

Slings the psychrometer for at least a minute but not more than one minute and a half ❑ Yes ❑ No

Reads the dry thermometer ❑ Yes ❑ No

Reads the wet thermometer ❑ Yes ❑ No

Reports humidity correctly ❑ Yes ❑ No

Completes task in five minutes or less

Passing-point total: 4

Reference: 8, pp. 69-70; 13, pp. 140-141

4. Vision Screening.

Places the athlete facing chart 20 feet away ❑ Yes ❑ No

Places athlete at the same level as chart ❑ Yes ❑ No

Has athlete read chart with left eye only ❑ Yes ❑ No

Has athlete cover right eye not being tested ❑ Yes ❑ No

Has athlete read chart with right eye only ❑ Yes ❑ No

Has athlete cover left eye not being tested ❑ Yes ❑ No
Has athlete read the smallest line on chart bilaterally ❑ Yes ❑ No
Completes task in five minutes or less

Passing-point total: 5

Reference: 1, pp. 9-10

5. Limb Girth Measurement.

Athlete is placed in supine position ❑ Yes ❑ No
Musculature of athlete is relaxed ❑ Yes ❑ No
Girth is measured at joint line ❑ Yes ❑ No
Girth is measured at least 10 centimeters proximal to joint line ❑ Yes ❑ No
Girth is measured at least 10 centimeters distal to joint line ❑ Yes ❑ No
Measure girth bilaterally at same sites ❑ Yes ❑ No
Measuring tape is wrinkle free ❑ Yes ❑ No
Completes task in five minutes or less

Passing-point total: 5

Reference: 13, p. 534

6. Postural Screening.

Positions athlete in a standing position ❑ Yes ❑ No
Plumb bob or pole is in alignment with anterior lateral malleolus ❑ Yes ❑ No
Checks the position of the plumb line in reference to the knee joint ❑ Yes ❑ No
Checks the position of the plumb line in reference to the greater trochanter ❑ Yes ❑ No
Checks the position of the plumb line in reference to the lumbar vertebrae ❑ Yes ❑ No
Checks the position of the plumb line in reference to the shoulder ❑ Yes ❑ No
Checks the position of the plumb line in reference to the cervical vertebrae ❑ Yes ❑ No
Checks the position of the plumb line in reference to the auditory meatus ❑ Yes ❑ No
Completes task in five minutes or less

Passing-point total: 6

Reference: 32, pp. 71-87

7. Cane Fitting.

Athlete positioned in a standing position ❑ Yes ❑ No

Athlete is wearing shoes ❑ Yes ❑ No

Measure from the greater trochanter to the floor ❑ Yes ❑ No

Selects the proper cane ❑ Yes ❑ No

Completes task in five minutes or less

Passing-point total: 3

Reference: 13, pp. 302-304

8. Deep Reflex Testing.

Places athlete supine or seated ❑ Yes ❑ No

Strokes the lateral plantar surface ❑ Yes ❑ No

Strokes the surface from heel to great toe ❑ Yes ❑ No

Completes task in five minutes or less

Passing-point total: 2

Reference: 29, p. 256

9. Fitting a Lateral Prophylactic Knee Brace. T

Places athlete in a standing position ❑ Yes ❑ No

Athlete's knee is bent 15 degrees ❑ Yes ❑ No

Places the brace on the lateral aspect of the knee ❑ Yes ❑ No

Neoprene top strap is strapped snugly ❑ Yes ❑ No

Hinge is in parallel lateral alignment with the axis of the knee ❑ Yes ❑ No

Hinge is (from an anterior view) in alignment with the joint line ❑ Yes ❑ No

Neoprene bottom strap is strapped snugly ❑ Yes ❑ No

Checks range of motion once brace is in place ❑ Yes ❑ No

Completes task in five minutes or less

Passing-point total: 6

Reference: 9, pp. 202-203

10. Use of Otoscope.

Places specula onto otoscope ❑ Yes ❑ No

Turns on the otoscope ❑ Yes ❑ No

Grasps the external ear and pulls posteriorly and superiorly ❑ Yes ❑ No

Inserts specula into ear canal ❑ Yes ❑ No

Looks into the otoscope ❑ Yes ❑ No

Holds otoscope with hand resting on athlete's cheek ❑ Yes ❑ No

Completes task in five minutes or less

Passing-point total: 4

Reference: 16, p. 83

11. PNF Contract Relax Stretching.

Positions athlete supine ❑ Yes ❑ No

Positions athlete near the edge of the table ❑ Yes ❑ No

Extends leg until tightness is felt ❑ Yes ❑ No

Athlete's knee is fully extended ❑ Yes ❑ No

Positions himself/herself to serve as resistance with lower leg resting on shoulder ❑ Yes ❑ No

Athlete contracts hamstring for six seconds ❑ Yes ❑ No

Does not allow movement during contraction ❑ Yes ❑ No

While in relaxed position maintains starting position ❑ Yes ❑ No

Athlete contracts quadriceps for six seconds ❑ Yes ❑ No

Resister moves thigh into more hip flexion ❑ Yes ❑ No

Repeats contract-relax at least three times ❑ Yes ❑ No

Completes task in five minutes or less

Passing-point total: 8

Reference: 44, pp. 7-8

12. Single Person Walking Assist.

Athlete's arm is placed over rescuer's neck/shoulder ❑ Yes ❑ No

Grasps athlete's hand (one that is over the neck) ❑ Yes ❑ No

Grasps athlete's waist at the opposite hip ❑ Yes ❑ No

Injured limb is next to rescuer's leg ❑ Yes ❑ No

Completes task in five minutes or less

Passing-point total: 3

Reference: 6, pp. 16-17; 23, pp. 646-647

13. Manual Muscle Testing of the Neck.

Muscle tests flexion ❑ Yes ❑ No

Resists neck flexion ❑ Yes ❑ No

Muscle tests extension ❑ Yes ❑ No

Resists neck extension ❑ Yes ❑ No

Muscle tests neck rotation to the right	❑ Yes	❑ No
Resists neck rotation to the right	❑ Yes	❑ No
Muscle tests neck rotation to the left	❑ Yes	❑ No
Resists neck rotation to the left	❑ Yes	❑ No
Muscle tests lateral flexion to the right	❑ Yes	❑ No
Resists lateral flexion to the right	❑ Yes	❑ No
Muscle tests lateral flexion to the left	❑ Yes	❑ No
Resists lateral flexion to the left	❑ Yes	❑ No
Completes task in five minutes or less		

Passing-point total: 8

Reference: 29, pp. 116-117; 32, pp. 318-319

14. Use of the Goniometer.

Stabilizes the metacarpal throughout testing	❑ Yes	❑ No
Goniometer placed on dorsal aspect of MCP (to test flexion) joint in alignment with longitudinal axis of phalanx	❑ Yes	❑ No
Axis of goniometer is over the MCP joint line	❑ Yes	❑ No
Bends all fingers during flexion	❑ Yes	❑ No
Goniometer placed on volar aspect of MCP (to test extension) joint in alignment with longitudinal axis of metacarpal	❑ Yes	❑ No
Axis of goniometer is over the MCP joint line	❑ Yes	❑ No
Finger is moved dorsal testing extension	❑ Yes	❑ No
Completes task in 10 minutes or less		

Passing-point total: 5

Reference: 19, p. 207

15. Testing the Cranial Nerves.

Athlete smells a pungent odor	❑ Yes	❑ No
Athlete read Snellen eye chart or identify an object	❑ Yes	❑ No
Athlete open eyelids wide and move the eye up, down, and toward the nose	❑ Yes	❑ No
Assesses athlete's sensitivity to touch on the face	❑ Yes	❑ No
Assesses athlete's mandible motion in depression, elevation, protrusion, and lateral deviation	❑ Yes	❑ No
Assesses athlete's ability to abduct eyes	❑ Yes	❑ No

Has athlete taste food ❑ Yes ❑ No

Assesses athlete's ability to protrude lips, close eyes, close mouth, move eyebrows, or dilate and constrict nasal passageways ❑ Yes ❑ No

Has athlete stand with eyes closed ❑ Yes ❑ No

Has athlete swallow ❑ Yes ❑ No

Assesses thoracic and abdominal viscera ❑ Yes ❑ No

Has athlete shrug shoulders and turn head ❑ Yes ❑ No

Has athlete stick out tongue ❑ Yes ❑ No

Completes task in five minutes or less

Passing-point total: 9

Reference: 38, pp. 3-20

16. Hip Adductor Strain Wrapping.

Athlete is in standing position with hip flexed about 20 degrees ❑ Yes ❑ No

Athlete internally rotates foot ❑ Yes ❑ No

Applies tape adherent ❑ Yes ❑ No

Applies elastic bandage from distal to proximal ❑ Yes ❑ No

Applies elastic bandage from lateral to medial ❑ Yes ❑ No

Elastic bandage is applied proximally around the waist, over the crest of the ilium ❑ Yes ❑ No

Applies a minimum of three overlapping white adhesive tape ❑ Yes ❑ No

Applies elastic bandage snugly ❑ Yes ❑ No

Elastic bandage is supportive ❑ Yes ❑ No

Completes task in three minutes or less

Passing-point total: 6

Reference: 66, pp. 64-65

17. Collateral Interphalangeal Joint Taping. T

Finger is positioned slightly flexed ❑ Yes ❑ No

Applies anchor strips distal and proximal to joint ❑ Yes ❑ No

Applies at least two strips in an x over each of the collateral aspects ❑ Yes ❑ No

Secures strips with closure tape ❑ Yes ❑ No

Taping is supportive ❑ Yes ❑ No

Tape is wrinkle free ❏ Yes ❏ No

Completes task in three minutes or less

Passing-point total: 4

Reference: 66, p. 113

18. Anterior Drawer Test.

Positions athlete in a supine position ❏ Yes ❏ No

Makes sure quadriceps and hamstrings are relaxed ❏ Yes ❏ No

Athlete's knee is flexed to 90 degrees ❏ Yes ❏ No

Athlete's foot is stabilized ❏ Yes ❏ No

Evaluator's hands are placed posteriorly on proximal tibia with thumbs on anterior joint line ❏ Yes ❏ No

Attempts to anteriorly displace tibia ❏ Yes ❏ No

Completes task in five minutes or less

Passing-point total: 4

Reference: 13, p. 529; 80, pp. 146-147

19. Apley's Compression Test.

Athlete is placed in a prone position ❏ Yes ❏ No

Athlete's knee is flexed to 90 degrees ❏ Yes ❏ No

Examiner places one hand on distal femur ❏ Yes ❏ No

Examiner places opposite hand on the plantar surface of foot ❏ Yes ❏ No

Tibia is compressed into the femur ❏ Yes ❏ No

Tibia is rotated internally on the femur ❏ Yes ❏ No

Tibia is rotated externally on the femur ❏ Yes ❏ No

Completes task in five minutes or less

Passing-point total: 5

Reference: 13, pp. 533-534; 29, pp. 191-193

20. Four-Way Straight Leg Raising.

Positions athlete lying down ❏ Yes ❏ No

Demonstrates forward flexion of hip with knee fully extended ❏ Yes ❏ No

Demonstrates abduction of hip with knee fully extended ❏ Yes ❏ No

Demonstrates extension of hip with knee fully extended ❏ Yes ❏ No

Demonstrates adduction of hip with knee fully extended ❑ Yes ❑ No

Completes task in five minutes or less

Passing-point total: 4

Reference: 24, p. 115; 85, pp. 91-94; 70, pp. 413-414, 448

21. Thomas Test.

Has athlete in supine position ❑ Yes ❑ No

Has athlete bring uninvolved knee into flexion ❑ Yes ❑ No

Stabilizes the pelvis ❑ Yes ❑ No

Has athlete complete active hip flexion ❑ Yes ❑ No

Applies resistance to hip flexion ❑ Yes ❑ No

Completes task in five minutes or less

Passing-point total: 4

Reference: 29, pp. 155-156

22. Trendelenburg Test.

Positions patient in a standing position both legs on the floor ❑ Yes ❑ No

Demonstrates that the pelvis is level prior to test ❑ Yes ❑ No

Has athlete stand on one leg ❑ Yes ❑ No

Checks level of pelvis ❑ Yes ❑ No

Completes task in five minutes or less

Passing-point total: 3

Reference: 38, pp. 178-180

23. Codman Pendulum Shoulder Exercises.

Stabilizes athlete at 45-90 degrees at the waist ❑ Yes ❑ No

Demonstrates horizontal (side to side) swinging of the arm ❑ Yes ❑ No

Demonstrates vertical (back and forth) swinging of the arm ❑ Yes ❑ No

Demonstrates clockwise swinging of the arm ❑ Yes ❑ No

Demonstrates counterclockwise swinging of the arm ❑ Yes ❑ No

Completes task in five minutes or less

Passing-point total: 4

Reference: 85, pp. 175-176

24. Apprehension Test of the Shoulder.

Abducts the arm/shoulder to at least 90 degrees ❑ Yes ❑ No

Fully externally rotates arm/shoulder ❑ Yes ❑ No

Checks athlete for expression of apprehension ❑ Yes ❑ No

Completes task in five minutes or less

Passing-point total: 2

Reference: 38, p. 61

25. Range of Motion of the Cervical Spine.

Demonstrates flexion of the cervical spine ❑ Yes ❑ No

Demonstrates extension of the cervical spine ❑ Yes ❑ No

Demonstrates rotation right of the cervical spine ❑ Yes ❑ No

Demonstrates rotation left of the cervical spine ❑ Yes ❑ No

Demonstrates lateral bending right of the cervical spine ❑ Yes ❑ No

Demonstrates lateral bending left of the cervical spine ❑ Yes ❑ No

Completes task in five minutes or less

Passing-point total: 4

Reference: 19, pp. 64-66; 80, p. 269

26. Louisiana Ankle Wrap.

Applied over a sock ❑ Yes ❑ No

Ankle is placed in neutral position ❑ Yes ❑ No

Two heel locks applied ❑ Yes ❑ No

Two figure of eight applied ❑ Yes ❑ No

Wrap is wrinkle free ❑ Yes ❑ No

Tape support is applied over wrap and proximally to sock ❑ Yes ❑ No

Wrap is supportive ❑ Yes ❑ No

Task is completed in three minutes or less

Passing-point total: 5

Reference: 66, p. 21

27. Thumb Check Rein for Hyperextension.

Positions thumb parallel to index finger ❑ Yes ❑ No

Applies a tape strip encircling thumb to index finger ❑ Yes ❑ No

Applies a strip of tape at the midpoint of encircling tape strip ❑ Yes ❑ No

Tape is supportive ❑ Yes ❑ No

Tape is wrinkle free ❑ Yes ❑ No

Completes task in three minutes or less

Passing-point total: 4

Reference: 13, p. 210

28. Metatarsal Arch Pad Application.

Applies tape adherent ❑ Yes ❑ No

Demonstrates cutting and beveling felt to size of metatarsal arch ❑ Yes ❑ No

Places beveled edge toward plantar surface ❑ Yes ❑ No

Demonstrates application of felt pad just proximal to second and fourth metatarsal heads ❑ Yes ❑ No

Demonstrates application of closure strips ❑ Yes ❑ No

Tape is wrinkle free ❑ Yes ❑ No

Pad is supportive ❑ Yes ❑ No

Completes task in three minutes or less

Passing-point total: 5

Reference: 66, p. 34

29. Glenohumeral Glide.

Athlete is supine ❑ Yes ❑ No

Athlete's arm is relaxed at his side ❑ Yes ❑ No

Distraction is applied lengthwise ❑ Yes ❑ No

Humeral head is moved anteriorally ❑ Yes ❑ No

Humeral head is moved posteriorlly ❑ Yes ❑ No

Completes task in five minutes or less

Passing-point total: 4

Reference: 10, pp. 162-163

30. Open Basket Weave.

Applies tape adherent ❑ Yes ❑ No

Applies heel pad to Achilles tendon area ❑ Yes ❑ No

Applies horseshoe to the lateral aspect of ankle ❑ Yes ❑ No

Applies an anchor at the mid-calf and just proximal to ball of foot ❑ Yes ❑ No

Foot is placed in neutral ❑ Yes ❑ No

Applies at least three stirrups—medial to lateral ❑ Yes ❑ No
Applies at least three horseshoe strips ❑ Yes ❑ No
Leaves the anterior aspect of ankle open ❑ Yes ❑ No
Applies overlapping strips up the stirrups ❑ Yes ❑ No
Applies locking strips anteriorly ❑ Yes ❑ No
Tape is wrinkle free ❑ Yes ❑ No
Completes task in three minutes or less

Passing-point total: 8:

Reference: 66, pp. 23-24

31. Great Toe Sprain Taping.

Applies tape adherent ❑ Yes ❑ No
Applies at least two figure of eight strips around the great toe ❑ Yes ❑ No
Applies at least two supporting strips lateral to medial ❑ Yes ❑ No
Applies locking or closure strip over ends of tape ❑ Yes ❑ No
Tape is supportive ❑ Yes ❑ No
Tape is wrinkle free ❑ Yes ❑ No
Completes task in three minutes or less

Passing-point total: 4

Reference: 66, pp. 35-36

32. Application of Immobilizer of the Knee (Postinjury).

Applies knee immobilizer with straps snug ❑ Yes ❑ No
Does not apply immobilizer strap over site of injury ❑ Yes ❑ No
Opening of immobilizer is in alignment with joint line and patella ❑ Yes ❑ No
Immobilizer is supportive ❑ Yes ❑ No
Immobilizer does not shift with gravity ❑ Yes ❑ No
Completes task in three minutes or less

Passing-point total: 4

Reference: 8, p. 204; 13, p. 560

33. Hamstring Strain Wrapping.

Athlete is in standing position ❑ Yes ❑ No
Athlete's knee is bent to fifteen degrees ❑ Yes ❑ No

Applies tape adherent ❑ Yes ❑ No

Applies elastic bandage from distal to proximal ❑ Yes ❑ No

Applies a minimum of three overlapping white adhesive tape ❑ Yes ❑ No

Applies elastic bandage snugly ❑ Yes ❑ No

Wrap is supportive ❑ Yes ❑ No

Task is completed in three minutes or less

Passing-point total: 5

Reference: 66, p. 68

34. Knee Pressure Wrapping for Acute Injury.

Applies wrap distal to proximal ❑ Yes ❑ No

Applies a compression pad over injury site ❑ Yes ❑ No

Applies wrap with more compress distally, less compression proximally ❑ Yes ❑ No

Overlaps wrap; by one half with each circle of wrap ❑ Yes ❑ No

Checks distal circulation upon completion ❑ Yes ❑ No

Wrap is wrinkle free ❑ Yes ❑ No

Completes task in three minutes or less

Passing-point total: 4

Reference: 2, p. 778; 8, pp. 142-143

35. Blister Padding.

Demonstrates beveling of the padding ❑ Yes ❑ No

Demonstrates padding goes completely around blister not on the blister itself ❑ Yes ❑ No

Demonstrates application of tape adherent ❑ Yes ❑ No

Taping is wrinkle free ❑ Yes ❑ No

Completes task in three minutes or less

Passing-point total: 3

Reference: 13, p. 822; 87, p. 750

36. Glenohumeral Joint Spica Wrap.

Positions athlete with arm internally rotated ❑ Yes ❑ No

Applies elastic bandage around upper arm and then encircling the chest ❑ Yes ❑ No

Wrap is applied in an internal rotation or toward the midline of body ❑ Yes ❑ No

Wrap covers the joint completely ❑ Yes ❑ No

Has athlete maintain slight expansion of chest ❑ Yes ❑ No

Traces wrap with tape ❑ Yes ❑ No

Elastic bandage is supportive decreasing abduction and external rotation ❑ Yes ❑ No

Complete task in three minutes or less

Passing-point total: 5

Reference: 66, pp. 81-82

37. Elbow Epicondylitis Taping.

Positions arm in pronation ❑ Yes ❑ No

Applies tape adherent ❑ Yes ❑ No

Applies felt pad over affected area ❑ Yes ❑ No

Encircles pad to hold in place ❑ Yes ❑ No

Tape is supportive ❑ Yes ❑ No

Tape is wrinkle free ❑ Yes ❑ No

Completes task in three minutes or less

Passing-point total: 4

Reference: 66, p.95

38. Acromioclavicular Joint Contusion Padding.

Positions athlete with hand on hip and chest expanded ❑ Yes ❑ No

Applies Band-Aid to nipple ❑ Yes ❑ No

Applies tape adherent ❑ Yes ❑ No

Applies horizontal anchor from anterior to posterior over distal ribs ❑ Yes ❑ No

Applies at least three overlapping tape strips from superior shoulder to anchor ❑ Yes ❑ No

Constructs a donut pad ❑ Yes ❑ No

Applies donut pad over the acromioclavicular joint ❑ Yes ❑ No

Applies closure strips encircling torso ❑ Yes ❑ No

Tape is supportive ❑ Yes ❑ No

Tape is wrinkle free ❑ Yes ❑ No

Completes task in three minutes or less

Passing-point total: 7

Reference: 66, pp. 76-78

C
APPENDIX

Answers to the Written Simulation Study Questions

When taking the written simulation, you'll mark your answer or answers with a highlight pen, and you will receive immediate feedback on whether your response is correct or not. What follows is a list of the feedback you'll receive for each possible response you choose for each item in chapter 8. To benefit most from this section, have a partner read aloud the feedback as you select your responses. For instance, for Problem 1 in chapter 8, if you select #4, "Visually check the athlete's body position," as an appropriate response to the scenario described, you would say aloud, "Number 4: Visually check the athlete's body position." Your partner would then read the feedback for #4: "Athlete is being held up by two teammates and being walked around." Taking into consideration the feedback you have received from your partner, you would then proceed to the next response you would make in the scenario described. Passing point totals are 70% of total points possible.

Problem 1

1. She says she finished the race about three minutes ago and that she feels weak, exhausted, and nauseous; she'd like a drink of water. ++
2. Inappropriate. – –
3. Not necessary. 0
4. Athlete is being held up by two teammates and being walked around. ++
5. Not necessary. 0
6. Athlete is conscious. ++
7. Inappropriate. – –
8. She indicates she has no medical conditions. ++
9. Athlete has no pain. ++
10. Athlete is pale and slightly sweaty. ++
11. She says no. ++

What you know: There is a pale, sweaty conscious athlete at the finish line of a cross country meet. ***Priorities:*** Determine the extent of the athlete's injury or illness.

12. Inappropriate. – –
13. It's normal. 0
14. Nothing found. ++
15. She says she's not. ++
16. She had half a glass of pop. ++
17. It is 95 and weak. ++
18. Rate is 24 per minute. ++
19. She says she had a 2,500-calorie meal about four hours earlier. ++
20. Inappropriate. – –
21. Blood pressure is 100/75. ++

What you know: The athlete has a rapid weak pulse with little fluid intake. ***Priorities:*** Continue to determine the cause of the illness.

22. Breath sounds are clear. 0
23. Inappropriate. Athlete goes into cardiac arrest and dies. Go to the next question. – –
24. Appropriate. ++
25. Inappropriate. – –
26. Inappropriate. – –
27. Inappropriate. – –
28. Inappropriate. – –
29. Inappropriate. – –
30. Inappropriate. – –
31. Inappropriate. – –
32. Inappropriate. – –
33. Athlete's status does not change. 0
34. Inappropriate. – –
35. Inappropriate. – –
36. Inappropriate. – –
37. Athlete begins to show improvement. ++
38. Inappropriate. Go to next question. – –
39. Inappropriate. – –
40. Inappropriate. – –

What you know: The athlete has improved with drinking of fluids. ***Priorities:*** Determine the illness.

41. Inappropriate. – –
42. Inappropriate. – –
43. Inappropriate. – –
44. Inappropriate. – –
45. Yes: good work. ++
46. Inappropriate. – –
47. Inappropriate. – –
48. Inappropriate. – –
49. Inappropriate. – –
50. Inappropriate. – –
51. Inappropriate. – –

What you know: Athlete is dehydrated. ***Priorities:*** Prevention of dehydration in the future.

52. Incorrect. – –
53. Incorrect. – –
54. Incorrect. – –
55. Incorrect. – –
56. Good idea. ++
57. Incorrect. – –
58. Good idea. ++
59. Good idea. ++
60. Incorrect. – –
61. Incorrect. – –
62. Incorrect. – –
63. Good idea. ++

What you know: There is a plan to prevent dehydration. ***Priorities:*** Distribute the plan and educate others. ***Passing-point total:*** 29

Problem 2

1. He does not respond. 0
2. Athlete is now face down. – –
3. He does not respond. ++
4. Inappropriate. – –
5. Athlete is lying supine, and the scene is safe. ++
6. Athlete breathes normally. ++
7. Unnecessary at this time. –
8. It's normal. ++
9. Nobody knows. ++
10. Airway is closed. ++
11. Airway is opened, but breathing is obstructed. ++
12. This exacerbates the injury. – –
13. Athlete having difficulty breathing. ++
14. Inappropriate. – –
15. Inappropriate. – –
16. The other team's athletic trainers asks if she can help. ++
17. They are on the way. ++

What you know: An unconscious injured athlete who is breathing and has a heartbeat, with an ambulance on the way. ***Priorities:*** Determine all injuries and illnesses prior to the arrival of the ambulance.

18. Inappropriate. – –
19. Inappropriate. – –
20. Appropriate. No obvious injuries are found; athlete remains unconscious going on three minutes. ++
21. Rate is 12 per minute. ++
22. Inappropriate. – –
23. Inappropriate. – –
24. Helmet is securely in place; the opposing teams' athletic trainer assists you. ++
25. Rate and quality are normal. ++
26. Inappropriate. – –
27. Appropriate; no medical conditions listed. ++
28. It's normal. ++
29. Pupils are unequal. ++
30. No severe bleeding. ++
31. None found. 0

What you know: An unconscious athlete has no obvious injuries or illnesses; you suspect a head or spinal cord injury. ***Priorities:*** Give care to prevent compromise of the airway, breathing, and circulation or paralysis.

32. Inappropriate. – –
33. All are normal. +
34. Inappropriate. – –
35. No deformities noted. +
36. No deformities noted. +
37. Inappropriate. – –
38. Not possible to do. – –
39. No deformities noted. +
40. Both are normal. +
41. They are normal. +
42. No deformities noted. +
43. Not necessary at this time. –
44. No deformities noted. +
45. Normal. +

What you know: Suspect head and/or neck injury. ***Priorities:*** Stabilize the athlete's condition, while determining other injuries. Monitor vital signs.

46. Seizure resolves. ++
47. Appropriate. ++
48. It's clear. ++
49. Unobstructed. +
50. Appropriate. ++
51. Athlete has a grand mal seizure; it lasts for one and a half minutes. ++
52. Not necessary at this time. –
53. Pupils dilate, but this does not change the situation. – –
54. Inappropriate. – –
55. Appropriate. ++
56. Helpful. ++
57. Not necessary. – –
58. Helpful. ++
59. Appropriate. ++
60. Helpful. ++
61. Helpful. ++
62. Helpful. ++

What you know: Athlete has a serious head injury. The seizure likely a sign of the head injury. ***Priorities:*** Get the athlete to the hospital, and treat for shock.

63. Inappropriate. – –
64. Inappropriate. – –
65. Inappropriate. – –
66. Inappropriate. – –
67. Inappropriate. – –
68. Inappropriate. – –
69. Appropriate. ++
70. Appropriate. ++
71. Appropriate. ++

What you know: Athlete is seriously injured requiring immediate hospitalization. Life is dependent upon getting to the hospital as soon as possible. ***Priorities:*** Get the athlete to the hospital and contact the family. ***Passing-point total:*** 51

Problem 3

1. She has circulation. 0
2. It's open. 0
3. Unnecessary at this time. –
4. Unnecessary. – –
5. None seen. +
6. Inappropriate. – –
7. It is. Athlete is lying supine. +
8. Appropriate. ++
9. She says everything but her neck. ++
10. She is conscious and complaining. +

11. Unnecessary. – –
12. Inappropriate. – –
13. Don't find one. 0
14. Not necessary at this time. –
15. Says everyone ran over her and she hurts everywhere but her neck and that she's tired. +
16. She's breathing. 0

What you know: Athlete is supine, everything hurts except for her neck. ***Priorities:*** Determine the nature of injury or illness.

17. 118 over 78. ++
18. Not necessary at this time. –
19. Pulse is rapid and weak. ++
20. Inappropriate. – –
21. Athlete gags and rips it out of her mouth. – –
22. Inappropriate. – –
23. Not necessary at this time. 0
24. Inappropriate. – –
25. Not necessary. – –
26. Inappropriate. – –
27. She says she does not. 0
28. 20 per minute. ++
29. Not necessary. – –
30. Inappropriate. – –

What you know: Athlete has a rapid weak pulse and an increased respiratory rate. ***Priorities:*** Determine the nature of illness or injury.

31. Her head snaps backward and eyes dilate) – –
32. She says she had chicken pox as a child and she has been tired lately; athlete seems confused. ++
33. She says she hears you fine. –
34. She says she has none. +
35. She has her balance. –
36. Not helpful. –
37. Inappropriate. – –
38. She says she takes nothing. +
39. She says it's just sore but more than anything she is tired. ++
40. Not necessary. –
41. It's on the way. ++

What you know: Athlete is tired. ***Priorities:*** Determine the nature of illness or injury.

42. Inappropriate. – –
43. Inappropriate. – –
44. Skin is warm and dry. ++
45. No bleeding or deformities noted. ++
46. She says no. 0
47. None found. 0
48. Inappropriate. – –
49. Inappropriate. – –
50. Pupils equal and reactive; eyes appear to be sunken. ++
51. No fluids or deformities noted. ++
52. No fluids or deformities noted. ++
53. No fluids or deformities noted. ++
54. Inappropriate. – –
55. No bleeding or deformities noted. ++
56. No fluids or deformities noted. ++
57. Athlete's breath smells of acetone, but there's no bleeding or deformities noted; athlete appears confused. ++
58. No bleeding or deformities noted. ++
59. Normal; athlete is embarrassed. 0
60. She says she has not eaten today; she says she feels dizzy and then vomits. ++
61. No bleeding or deformities noted. ++
62. Okay, no change occurs. 0
63. She says no. 0
64. She says okay, but she's getting more tired by the minute. +

What you know: Athlete has an acetone breath, she is confused, tired, and she has not eaten. ***Priorities:*** Treat the cause of illness.

65. Not necessary. – –
66. Not necessary. – –
67. Heart rate is 90 per minute. ++
68. She feels a little better; paramedics take her to the hospital. ++
69. Athlete pushes you away. – –
70. Not necessary. – –
71. Not necessary. – –
72. Not necessary. –
73. She's confused by what's going on. +
74. Inappropriate. – –
75. Helpful. +
76. Not necessary. – –
77. Helpful. +
78. Not necessary. – –
79. Athlete dies. Go to next question. – –
80. Not necessary. – –

What you know: Athlete feels better after eating. ***Priorities:*** Determine illness based on signs and symptoms.

81. Incorrect. – –
82. Incorrect. – –
83. Incorrect. – –
84. Correct. ++
85. Incorrect. – –
86. Incorrect. – –
87. Incorrect. – –
88. Incorrect. – –
89. Incorrect. – –

What you know: Athlete has diabetic illness. ***Priorities:*** Prevent reoccurrence.

90. Excellent. ++
91. Excellent idea. ++
92. Inappropriate. – –
93. Inappropriate. – –
94. Inappropriate. – –
95. Inappropriate. – –
96. Inappropriate. – –
97. Inappropriate. – –
98. Inappropriate. – –
99. Inappropriate. – –
100. Inappropriate. – –
101. Excellent. ++
102. Inappropriate. – –
103. Excellent. ++

What you know: Athlete needs to eat to accommodate exercise. ***Priorities:*** Implement plan and refer athlete to physician for care. ***Passing-point total:*** 45

Problem 4

1. You know the way. 0
2. Inappropriate at this time. – –
3. They don't know the athlete. 0
4. Inappropriate. – –
5. Appropriate. ++
6. Inappropriate. – –
7. Appropriate. ++
8. They do not calm down and tell you to hurry. –
9. Inappropriate. – –
10. They do not know the athlete. –
11. They continue to tell you to hurry. 0
12. Inappropriate. – –
13. Inappropriate. – –
14. Inappropriate. – –
15. It's cold. 0
16. Inappropriate. – –
17. It delays care. – –

What you know: Athlete is injured on the track. ***Priorities:*** Get to the athlete and determine extent of injury.

18. Air goes into the lungs. ++
19. Okay, no changes occur. ++
20. Another athlete arrives, and you send her to call for an ambulance. ++
21. There's no pulse. ++
22. Athlete is lying on his left side; he has singed hair with no other apparent injuries. ++
23. They indicate he was running and collapsed after being hit by lightning. ++
24. Not necessary at this time. –
25. Athlete does not respond. ++
26. Athlete is now supine. ++
27. Not necessary. –
28. Appropriate. ++
29. Unnecessary. – –
30. Unnecessary. – –
31. Athlete is not breathing. ++
32. Appropriate. ++

What you know: An athlete has been hit by lightning. He has no breathing or heartbeat. ***Priorities:*** Give CPR until paramedics arrive.

33. Inappropriate. – –
34. Inappropriate. – –
35. Inappropriate. – –
36. Inappropriate; there is none. – –
37. Appropriate. ++
38. Inappropriate. – –
39. Inappropriate. – –
40. You have found the xiphoid process. ++
41. Inappropriate. – –
42. Inappropriate. – –
43. Air does not make the chest rise. ++
44. Inappropriate. – –
45. Inappropriate. – –
46. Appropriate. ++
47. Appropriate. ++
48. Inappropriate. – –

49. Your breaths go in. ++
50. Inappropriate. – –
51. Appropriate. ++
52. Inappropriate. – –
53. Inappropriate. – –

What you know: Athlete has no breathing or heartbeat. ***Priorities:*** Continue CPR.

54. Inappropriate. – –
55. Inappropriate. – –
56. Inappropriate. – –
57. Inappropriate. – –
58. Inappropriate. – –
59. Inappropriate. – –
60. Whom are you doing this with? – –
61. Inappropriate. – –
62. Appropriate. (The paramedics load the athlete and transport him to the hospital) ++
63. Inappropriate. – –
64. Unnecessary. – –

What you know: Athlete requires immediate attention by a physician and has been taken to the hospital. ***Priorities:*** Get parents to hospital and document injury.

65. Inappropriate. – –
66. Inappropriate. – –
67. Inappropriate. – –
68. Inappropriate. – –
69. Inappropriate. – –
70. Inappropriate. – –
71. Helpful. +
72. He does not know. 0
73. Inappropriate. – –
74. Inappropriate. – –
75. They go to the hospital. +

What you know: Parents are headed to hospital and you have documented injury. ***Priorities:*** Prevent further injury from lightning.

76. Inappropriate. – –
77. Appropriate. ++
78. Appropriate. ++
79. Inappropriate. – –
80. Good idea. ++
81. Inappropriate. – –
82. Inappropriate. – –
83. Appropriate. ++
84. Inappropriate. – –
85. Inappropriate. – –
86. Inappropriate. – –

What you know: You have a plan to prevent lightning injury. ***Priorities:*** Put plan into place.
Passing-point total: 32

Problem 5

1. He is. +
2. Good choice. ++
3. Not helpful. – –
4. It's open. 0
5. Not necessary at this time. –
6. He takes it and applies it to his face, which is pouring blood; his arms are saturated in blood, and he says he feels light headed ++
7. It is. 0
8. He does. +
9. Seconds before. 0
10. The athlete says he was playing catch in the hallway, dove, and fell through a glass door. +
11. Appropriate. ++

What you know: An athlete has severe bleeding laceration of both arms and face. The athlete feels light-headed. ***Priorities:*** Stop bleeding and prevent the athlete from passing out, while paramedics are called.

12. Bleeding appears to slow. ++
13. Does not help. –
14. The athlete is comfortable. ++
15. This does not seem to slow the blood flow. ++
16. They are on the way; however, the student says he does not feel well and breaks his fall passing out onto the floor. ++
17. The athlete reports he is light headed. +
18. He does not respond. +
19. The athlete's arms begin to gush blood again. – –
20. The student says he does not feel well. 0
21. This is helpful. ++
22. Nothing appears abnormal; his chest expands with each breath. ++

23. Not helpful. – –
24. Not helpful. – –
25. Not helpful. – –
26. Not helpful. – –
27. Not helpful. – –
28. Not applicable. – –
29. He has normal skin color. +

What you know: You are attempting to control bleeding and prevent athlete from passing out. The student is passed out but has no visual injuries. The student is breathing. ***Priorities:*** Control bleeding of the athlete and treat for shock.

30. He feels light headed and lays back down. –
31. Why? – –
32. The bleeding subsides. ++
33. Inappropriate. – –
34. Unnecessary. – –
35. Okay. +
36. Unnecessary. – –
37. Bleeding appears to slow. ++
38. Unnecessary at this time. – –
39. Unnecessary. – –
40. Helpful. +

What you know: Bleeding is controlled and shock care is in place for the athlete. ***Priorities:*** Treat the student.

41. He is breathing. +
42. Unnecessary at this time. 0
43. Unnecessary. – –
44. Unnecessary. – –
45. Unnecessary. – –
46. Unnecessary. – –
47. Inappropriate. – –
48. He says he has none. ++
49. Unnecessary. – –
50. Unnecessary. – –
51. Airway is open. +
52. Inappropriate. – –
53. He has circulation. +
54. He says he felt light-headed upon seeing the blood. ++
55. He says he's doing fine; bleeding is controlled. ++
56. Inappropriate. – –
57. Inappropriate. – –
58. Inappropriate. – –
59. None was found. – –
60. He has a bump on the back of his head. +
61. He is starting to become coherent. ++
62. He has a headache and some pain at the back of his head. +

What you know: The student has airway, breathing and circulation, and a bump on his head. ***Priorities:*** Treat the student for shock.

63. Unnecessary. – –
64. Unnecessary. – –
65. Unnecessary. – –
66. Unnecessary. – –
67. Student is now cold but it does not make him feel better. – –
68. Good, he feels better. ++
69. Appropriate. +
70. Inappropriate. – –
71. It's painful but helpful; student says he's embarrassed to stand up and sits in a chair. ++
72. No change. 0
73. Inappropriate. – –
74. Inappropriate. – –

What you know: Student had a fainting spell. ***Priorities:*** Monitor both the athlete and student and await the ambulance.

75. Unnecessary. – –
76. Unnecessary. – –
77. Unnecessary. – –
78. It's comparable both sides, with a one-second refill. +
79. It's 104/72. ++
80. Unnecessary. – –
81. It's 60. ++

What you know: Athlete's blood pressure is low. ***Priorities:*** Get athlete to hospital for care.

82. Helpful. +
83. He is loaded into the ambulance. ++
84. Unnecessary. – –
85. Appropriate. ++
86. He refuses to go. +
87. They will meet the ambulance at the hospital. ++
88. Inappropriate. – –

89. Unnecessary. – –
90. Okay, they do not want to come in. +
91. Okay. +
92. Not needed but nice. 0
93. Okay. +
94. Unnecessary. – –

What you know: Make contact with family of the athlete and student. ***Priorities:*** Document injuries. ***Passing-point total:*** 43

Problem 6

1. Good idea. ++
2. Not helpful. – –
3. Inappropriate. – –
4. Inappropriate. – –
5. The area is safe; athlete is lying supine. ++
6. It is on the way. ++
7. Athlete does not respond. ++
8. Nobody is around. 0
9. There is a heartbeat. ++
10. Inappropriate. – –
11. Inappropriate. – –
12. It is open. ++
13. None seen. +
14. Inappropriate. – –
15. Athlete is breathing. ++
16. There is no bleeding. ++
17. Appropriate. ++

What you know: An athlete is injured and unconscious but has airway, breathing, and circulation. ***Priorities:*** Determine the nature of injury or illness while paramedics are on the way.

18. It is open. 0
19. It is rapid and weak. ++
20. Athlete is breathing. +
21. Not appropriate. – –
22. It is 118 over 78. ++
23. Skin color is normal. +
24. Not necessary. – –
25. Not necessary. – –
26. Not necessary at this time. _
27. Not helpful. – –
28. It is 12 per minute. ++
29. Athlete is now prone. – –
30. Appropriate. Athlete's eyes flutter and roll back. ++
31. None found and care is delayed. – –

What you know: Athlete appears normal but is unresponsive. ***Priorities:*** Do a secondary survey to determine nature of illness or injury.

32. No fluids or deformities noted. ++
33. Athlete chokes. – –
34. Athlete chokes. – –
35. Okay. Athlete is breathing and has a pulse. ++
36. Not in the scope of practice. – –
37. No change occurs. 0
38. Athlete's breath is normal. There is a saliva dripping down her cheek. ++
39. Not necessary. – –
40. Not necessary. – –
41. Not necessary. – –
42. No bleeding or deformities noted. ++
43. Not necessary. – –
44. No bleeding or deformities noted. ++
45. Saliva drains out of mouth. ++
46. Appropriate. No deformities or fluids found. ++
47. Inappropriate. – –
48. No bleeding or deformities noted. ++
49. Not necessary. – –
50. Appropriate. No deformities or fluids found. ++

What you know: No abnormal findings are found in the survey, but the athlete is still unconscious. ***Priorities:*** Continue secondary survey.

51. No deformities noted. ++
52. No fluids or deformities noted. ++
53. It remains normal. ++
54. No deformities noted. ++
55. Now you are in trouble for false alarm. – –
56. No deformities noted. ++
57. No deformities noted. ++
58. Inappropriate. – –
59. Breath sounds are equal and clear. ++

What you know: No abnormal findings are found in the survey, but the athlete is still unconscious. ***Priorities:*** Continue secondary survey.

60. No deformities noted. ++
61. Not necessary. – –
62. Urine noted, but no deformities noted. ++
63. No deformities noted. ++
64. You feel better but the athlete is unresponsive. – –
65. Not necessary. – –
66. Abdominal sounds are equal. ++
67. Inappropriate. – –
68. No deformities noted. ++
69. No reason to do this. – –
70. Inappropriate. – –
71. No deformities noted. ++
72. It is normal. ++
73. Not necessary. – –
74. Not necessary. – –
75. It is within normal limits. ++
76. Not necessary. – –
77. No deformities noted. ++
78. Not necessary. – –
79. Not necessary. – –
80. Nobody is around. –

What you know: No abnormal findings in the survey, but the athlete is still unconscious. ***Priorities:*** Continue secondary survey.

81. Not necessary. – –
82. Not necessary. – –
83. No deformities noted. ++
84. The abandonment of a patient is worthy of a lawsuit. – –
85. Both are within normal limits. ++
86. No deformities noted. ++
87. One second refill. ++
88. Inappropriate. – –
89. No deformities noted. ++
90. Not necessary. – –
91. Not necessary. – –
92. No deformities or fluids noted. ++
93. Inappropriate. – –
94. Pulse normal. ++
95. Inappropriate. – –
96. Helpful. ++
97. Normal response noted. ++
98. Appropriate. ++

What you know: No abnormal findings are found in the survey, but the athlete is still unconscious. ***Priorities:*** Continue secondary survey. Treat athlete for shock and get to the hospital.

99. No deformities noted. ++
100. There is no change. +
101. Pulse is regular at 60 per minute. ++
102. Helpful. ++
103. No deformities or fluids noted. ++
104. No deformities noted. ++
105. Good. +

What you know: Monitor the athlete. ***Priorities:*** Get athlete to hospital.

106. Okay. +
107. Excellent. ++
108. Good idea. ++
109. They will meet the athlete at the hospital. +
110. That will help. +
111. No camera is found. – –
112. Not helpful. – –

What you know: Athlete is on the way to the hospital. ***Priorities:*** Document and await referral from physician as to diagnosis. ***Passing-point total:*** 83

Problem 7

1. You are in the training room. – –
2. She is trying to stand. –
3. She says she stepped on someone's foot. ++
4. It is. – –
5. She says she has not hurt her ankle before. ++
6. She says on the lateral side of her ankle. ++
7. Not necessary. – –
8. Just a few seconds ago. ++
9. Not necessary. – –
10. She says no. ++
11. She says no. ++
12. It's normal. +
13. She says she felt it snap. ++
14. Not necessary. – –
15. No bleeding found. 0
16. She says it's painful. ++
17. Not necessary. – –

What you know: Athlete injured her ankle and has no previous history. ***Priorities:*** Determine the extent of the injury.

18. Not necessary. – –
19. Not necessary. – –
20. Not necessary. – –
21. It's too painful to walk. –
22. Not necessary. – –
23. There's a lateral golfball-sized lump. ++
24. Not necessary. – –
25. Not necessary. – –
26. There's a lateral golfball-sized lump. ++
27. None yet. +
28. Not necessary. – –

What you know: Athlete has a lateral lump on her ankle. ***Priorities:*** Determine if the injury is a fracture or sprain.

29. Not helpful. –
30. Not helpful. –
31. She says it does not hurt. ++
32. She says that's painful. ++
33. She says it is okay. +
34. Not necessary. – –
35. She says it's painful. ++
36. She says it doesn't hurt. +
37. No problem. 0
38. Nothing found. 0
39. She says it does not hurt. +
40. No problem. 0
41. Not helpful. –
42. She says this does not hurt. +
43. She says that it's painful. ++
44. She says it's not painful. +
45. She says it's fine. ++
46. Not necessary. – –
47. This is not painful. +
48. She says it's not painful. ++
49. She says it does not hurt. +
50. She says it does not hurt. +
51. Not helpful. –
52. Not necessary. – –
53. Not helpful. –
54. She says it does not hurt. ++
55. Not necessary. – –
56. Not necessary. – –

What you know: Athlete has an ankle sprain. ***Priorities:*** Perform special tests to determine extent of injury.

57. Not necessary. – –
58. Not appropriate at this time. 0
59. Not necessary. – –
60. Not necessary. – –
61. Not necessary. – –
62. It's normal. +
63. Not necessary. – –
64. Normal. +
65. Normal. +

What you know: Athlete likely has an ankle sprain with normal circulation. ***Priorities:*** Perform special tests to determine extent of injury.

66. Not necessary. –
67. Athlete has difficulty with dorsiflexion and inversion. ++
68. Not necessary. – –
69. Not necessary. – –
70. Athlete has difficulty with dorsiflexion and inversion. ++
71. Not necessary. – –
72. Athlete has difficulty with dorsiflexion and inversion. ++
73. She says it's too painful. +
74. She says that touching is now painful. +
75. Not necessary. –
76. She says that does not hurt. +
77. The test is negative. ++
78. All are normal. +
79. She says that it's painful. +

What you know: Athlete likely has an ankle sprain with decreased range of motion and pain. ***Priorities:*** Treat the injury.

80. It causes increased swelling from the bubbles. –
81. Excellent idea. ++
82. Good. ++
83. Athlete screams in pain. – –
84. The ankle enlarges. – –
85. Good idea. ++
86. The ankle enlarges. – –
87. Helpful. ++

What you know: Athlete likely has a lateral ankle sprain and cryotherapy helps. ***Priorities:*** Continue to decrease swelling and pain. Eventually increase range of motion and strength. Refer to physician if not better. ***Passing-point total:*** 47

Problem 8

1. He says he has no idea. ++
2. He noticed the problem a month ago but thought it would go away. ++
3. He says he has no pain. 0
4. He says no. – –
5. He says no. – –
6. He has not stopped. – –
7. Not necessary. – –
8. He says it is his lip. – –
9. He says no. 0
10. He says this is the first time he's seeking help. 0
11. Inappropriate. – –
12. Inappropriate. – –
13. Inappropriate. – –
14. Inappropriate. – –
15. He says sometimes his tongue is numb. ++
16. Inappropriate. – –
17. He says yes. ++
18. He says yes. ++
19. He says just a sore throat. ++
20. He says no. +

What you know: An athlete has a sore throat and a lump on his lip. ***Priorities:*** Determine the nature of illness or injury.

21. Inappropriate. – –
22. Inappropriate. – –
23. Inappropriate. – –
24. Inappropriate. – –
25. Inappropriate. – –
26. Inappropriate. – –
27. Raccoon eyes. – –
28. Inappropriate. – –
29. Inappropriate. – –
30. Inappropriate. – –
31. Inappropriate. – –
32. They're discolored in a brownish tone. ++
33. Inappropriate. – –
34. It has a white patch on the inside of his lip but nothing in his throat. ++
35. He says he chews tobacco. ++
36. Inappropriate. – –

What you know: Athlete uses chewing tobacco and may have an illness related to its use. ***Priorities:*** Determine the extent of the illness.

37. Inappropriate. – –
38. Inappropriate. – –
39. Inappropriate. – –
40. Inappropriate. – –
41. Inappropriate. – –
42. Inappropriate. – –
43. Inappropriate. – –
44. Nothing noted. ++
45. Nothing noted. ++
46. Nothing noted. ++
47. Nothing noted. ++
48. Some elevations felt. ++
49. Inappropriate. – –
50. Not necessary. – –

What you know: Has swollen glands. ***Priorities:*** Determine if the athlete has an infection or more serious illness.

51. It's 98.6 degrees Fahrenheit. +
52. He has wonderful vision, but it does not help this case. – –
53. Not necessary. – –
54. Not necessary. – –
55. Not necessary. – –
56. Not necessary. – –
57. Not necessary. – –
58. Not necessary. – –
59. Not necessary. – –
60. Not necessary. – –

What you know: Athlete may have lip cancer or some underlying illness. ***Priorities:*** Get the athlete to physician for extensive evaluation.

61. Appropriate. ++
62. Inappropriate. – –
63. Inappropriate. – –
64. Inappropriate. – –
65. Inappropriate. – –
66. Inappropriate. – –
67. Appropriate. ++
68. Inappropriate. – –
69. Inappropriate. – –
70. Inappropriate. – –
71. Inappropriate. – –
72. Okay. 0

What you know: Athlete will be seeing a physician. ***Priorities:*** Await results from physician. ***Passing-point total:*** 22

Problem 9

1. Not necessary at this time. –
2. He does not feel any better. +
3. He has a cut on his forehead, but his mother picked him up. 0
4. He says it's his pole vaulter's blood. 0
5. He says he may get AIDS. ++
6. He was taking down his pole and it hit him in the head. 0
7. He has a cut on his forehead, but his mother picked him up. 0
8. He says one of his athletes hit his head and was bleeding everywhere. He says that the coach has a cut on his hand and had no latex gloves when he helped the athlete. ++
9. Not necessary. – –

What you know: An anxious coach has had contact with an athlete's blood. ***Priorities:*** Determine the extent of contact and protect yourself.

10. Good choice. ++
11. He soaps his hands and scrubs with a hand brush. ++
12. Excellent idea. ++
13. Okay. +
14. Wound is now covered. ++
15. Coach is upset—it's his coaching shirt. –
16. Not necessary. – –
17. Good. +
18. Great. ++
19. Okay. +
20. If you need to. 0
21. Not necessary. –

What you know: The coach needs to be tested. ***Priorities:*** Clean up the training room and protect yourself and others from possible transmission.

22. It shows nothing out of the ordinary. 0
23. Things are cleaned. ++
24. Not necessary. – –
25. Things are cleaned. ++
26. Things are sealed. ++
27. Inappropriate. – –
28. Not necessary. – –
29. Not necessary. – –
30. Not necessary. – –

What you know: Clean the training room and dispose of biohazards. ***Priorities:*** Document the injury.

31. That will help establish good documentation. ++
32. That will help establish good documentation. ++
33. Not necessary. – –
34. Okay. +
35. Yes, he was upset. ++
36. That will help establish good documentation. ++
37. The source will not. ++
38. Not necessary at this time. – –
39. That will help establish good documentation. ++
40. That might be helpful. +
41. That will help establish good documentation. ++
42. That will help establish good documentation. ++
43. That might be helpful. +

What you know: Documentation is complete. ***Priorities:*** Develop an educational program to prevent transmission of blood-borne pathogens.

44. Good. ++
45. Good. ++
46. Good idea. ++
47. Good. ++
48. Okay. +
49. Good. +
50. Absolutely. ++
51. Good. ++
52. Okay. 0
53. Good. ++
54. Possibly. 0
55. Not helpful. –
56. Bad idea: you can get sued for invasion of privacy. – –
57. Bad idea: you can get sued for violating due to the disability act. – –

58. Good. ++
59. Good. ++
60. Good. ++
61. Bad idea: you can get sued for violating due to the disability act. – –
62. Bad idea: you can get sued for invasion of privacy. – –

What you know: You have a good program. ***Priorities:*** Educate staff and athletes. ***Passing-point total:*** 46

Problem 10

1. He says pain is constant. ++
2. He says he has no goals, and that the place would be better off without him. ++
3. Not necessary. – –
4. He says seven months ago. ++
5. Ask where was the pain initially. – –
6. He says hi. 0
7. He indicates he is always in severe pain. –
8. Not necessary. – –
9. Not necessary. – –
10. He says no. 0
11. He says none of the pain killers have helped: he is in constant pain. +
12. Inappropriate. – –
13. Not necessary. – –
14. He says no. 0
15. He responds by saying the opponent rotated his knee while his body was pinned to the mat. This athlete has the smell of alcohol on his breath. ++

What you know: You have an Olympic caliber athlete who has a knee injury that is so serious that he will not wrestle again. He smells of alcohol and has no goals. ***Priorities:*** Determine reason for alcohol use and lack of motivation.

16. Not necessary at this time. – –
17. He says, "Of course. What would you do if you couldn't wrestle again?" ++
18. Not necessary. – –
19. He says his wife divorced him. ++
20. He says he rarely eats, and he has lost his appetite. ++
21. Not necessary. – –
22. Not necessary. – –
23. Not necessary. – –
24. Not necessary. – –
25. Not necessary. – –
26. The scar show there have been multiple surgeries. 0
27. Not necessary. – –
28. Not necessary. – –
29. Not necessary. – –
30. Not necessary. – –
31. Not necessary. – –
32. He says he stays up and has difficulty sleeping. ++

What you know: Athlete has numerous losses. ***Priorities:*** Determine the athlete's mental health status.

33. "I thought about it on the way to therapy this morning." ++
34. Not necessary. – –
35. Not necessary. – –
36. Not necessary. – –
37. Not necessary. – –
38. Not necessary. – –
39. He says taking all the pills in the house. ++
40. Not necessary. – –
41. Not necessary. – –
42. Not necessary. – –
43. "Sure. I thought of driving my car into the bridge abutment." ++
44. He says, "My family is important. I really do not want to have to do anything." ++
45. Not necessary. – –
46. Not necessary. – –
47. He indicates he has a hunting rifle. ++
48. He says no, and that he is just ticked off right now. ++

What you know: Athlete is suicidal. ***Priorities:*** Get athlete to mental health care professional for assessment.

49. He says he has Blue Cross. +
50. Not necessary. – –
51. He says he just does not know. ++
52. Not necessary. – –

53. Not necessary. – –
54. Not necessary. – –
55. It may be helpful. +
56. He gives you his sister's phone number. ++
57. Not necessary. – –
58. Not necessary. – –
59. She says she will come and get him. ++
60. Not necessary. – –
61. He says he really does not care. He has heard the program before. 0
62. Not necessary. – –
63. Not necessary. – –
64. Not necessary. – –

What you know: Athlete is suicidal and requires care immediately. ***Priorities:*** Get someone to assist him by taking him to hospital. ***Passing-point total:*** 25

Problem 11

1. Unnecessary. – –
2. Okay. +
3. He says, "I'm in pain." 0
4. Athlete fights you. – –
5. He is conscious. –
6. Unnecessary at this time. –
7. He says no. +
8. The scene is safe. The athlete is rolling around on the field, face up. His left lower leg is displaced mid-shaft at 30 degrees. ++
9. Unnecessary at this time. –
10. The athlete is screaming in pain. +
11. Unnecessary. – –
12. Inappropriate. – –
13. Athlete is screaming in pain. –
14. Inappropriate. – –
15. Inappropriate. – –
16. Helmet is securely in place. – –
17. Okay. +

What you know: The injured athlete has a mid-shaft tibia fracture, but he refuses treatment. ***Priorities:*** Get permission to treat.

18. There is bleeding. ++
19. Bone slides beneath the skin. – –
20. They are on the way. +
21. He has circulation. +
22. Airway is open. +
23. He says no and then goes unconscious. ++
24. The athlete goes into shock. – –
25. He is breathing. +
26. Compound fracture worsens. – –

What you know: An unconscious athlete who has refused treatment has a compound displaced fracture. ***Priorities:*** Stop the bleeding, splint fracture, and prevent shock.

27. This helps the athlete. ++
28. This slows the bleeding. ++
29. This is not necessary. 0
30. This creates pain and destroys tissue. – –
31. Refill within two seconds. ++
32. That is helpful. ++
33. Not necessary. – –
34. This prevents some infection. ++
35. Not necessary at this time. –
36. The pain causes a groan from the athlete. –
37. Excellent. ++
38. This is not necessary. –

What you know: Bleeding has slowed, and you have partially treated for shock. ***Priorities:*** Continue to treat for shock and monitor vital signs.

39. The athlete goes deeper into shock. – –
40. This helps the athlete. ++
41. The athlete goes deeper into shock. – –
42. This helps the athlete. ++
43. Not helpful at this time. 0
44. Unnecessary. This is not in the scope of practice. – –
45. Breathing is rapid and shallow. ++
46. The rate is 28 per minute. ++
47. Excellent idea. ++
48. It is 130/96. ++

What you know: The athlete is in shock and requires physician's care. ***Priorities:*** Get athlete to the hospital. ***Passing-point total:*** 27

Problem 12

1. Flexion is 20 degrees, and there is full extension. ++
2. Strength is limited. +
3. It is eight inches. ++
4. The injured thigh has one inch greater girth. ++
5. Athlete indicates it is limited when immobilized. ++
6. All hip motions are limited by pain. ++
7. He cannot walk. –
8. It is eight inches. +

What you know: An athlete has thigh contusion. ***Priorities:*** Reduce the diameter of swelling.

9. Okay. ++
10. Okay. +
11. Okay. After three days the contusion decreases. ++
12. Not necessary. – –
13. Okay. ++
14. This creates pain. –
15. Inappropriate. –
16. Okay. +

What you know: Swelling is decreasing. ***Priorities:*** Increase range of motion.

17. Helpful. ++
18. Helpful. ++
19. Helpful. ++
20. Flexion is now to 45 degrees after three days. ++
21. Appropriate. ++
22. Appropriate. ++
23. Inappropriate. – –

What you know: Increase range of motion. ***Priorities:*** Increase strength.

24. Improvement is slow. ++
25. Improvement is good. ++
26. Not appropriate. – –
27. Strength is going well. ++
28. Range and strength are 80 percent of normal. ++
29. Athlete falls down in pain. – –
30. Appropriate. ++
31. Okay. After a week he has full range of motion. ++
32. Appropriate. ++
33. Appropriate. ++
34. This athlete says he cannot swim. 0
35. Athlete has no problems with exercise. ++

What you know: Strength is increasing, there is full range of motion. ***Priorities:*** Begin light drills.

36. Appropriate. ++
37. Appropriate. ++
38. Appropriate. ++
39. Appropriate. Athlete has 90 percent strength. ++
40. Appropriate. ++
41. Appropriate. ++
42. Appropriate. ++

What you know: Athlete has almost full strength. ***Priorities:*** Begin balance and sport-specific skills.

43. Not necessary. –
44. Okay. +
45. Appropriate. Athlete has 100 percent strength. ++
46. Appropriate. ++
47. Athlete is excited to play. ++
48. Appropriate. ++
49. Good. ++
50. Okay. +
51. Okay. +
52. Okay. +
53. Okay. +
54. Not helpful. –
55. Good. ++

What you know: Athlete has full strength. ***Priorities:*** Return athlete to practice.

56. Athlete feels stronger than ever before. ++
57. Athlete says he would play better without it, but he will try it your way. ++
58. Does not help. –
59. This is protective. ++
60. Coach is elated. +
61. Does not help. –

What you know: Athlete has full strength and range of motion. ***Priorities:*** Monitor athlete periodically. ***Passing-point total:*** 62

Problem 13

1. She asks you why you are asking as you took care of this initially. –
2. She asks you why you are asking as you took care of this initially. –
3. She asks you why you are asking as you took care of this initially. –
4. She asks you why you are asking as you took care of this initially. –
5. She asks you why you are asking as you took care of this initially. –
6. Not necessary. –
7. She asks you why you are asking as you took care of this initially. –
8. "Not now," she says. ++
9. She says she is not in pain. +
10. She asks you why you are asking as you took care of this initially. –
11. Not necessary. – –
12. Not necessary. – –
13. She says she wants to return to gymnastics. ++

What you know: A gymnast with a medial collateral ligament sprain of her elbow has decreased range of motion. ***Priorities:*** Assess the gymnast.

14. Not necessary. – –
15. None found. +
16. None found. +
17. None found. +
18. None found. +
19. None found. +
20. None found. +
21. The previously casted arm is smaller than the other. ++
22. None found. +
23. The previously casted arm is smaller than the other. ++

What you know: Athlete has decreased girth and swelling. ***Priorities:*** Determine the range of motion and stability of the joint.

24. The ligament is stable. ++
25. Unnecessary. – –
26. It is normal. +
27. It is normal. ++
28. The ligament is stable. +
29. Not necessary. 0
30. The range is 0 - 120 degrees. ++
31. The range is 0 - 80 degrees. ++
32. There is a light decrease in wrist pronators, biceps, triceps and wrist flexors. ++
33. The range is 0 - 20 degrees. +
34. The range is 0 - 30 degrees. ++
35. It is normal. +
36. It is normal. ++

What you know: Athlete has decreased range of motion but a stable joint. ***Priorities:*** Increase range of motion.

37. It is cold. +
38. Athlete has pain while doing this. –
39. Not appropriate at this time. –
40. Not appropriate at this time. –
41. Athlete has range up to 120 degrees of flexion. ++
42. Athlete has range from five to 120 degrees. ++
43. Appropriate. +
44. Good. ++
45. Athlete is able to get full wrist pronation. ++
46. Athlete is able to get full wrist pronation. ++
47. Appropriate. ++
48. Appropriate. ++
49. Appropriate. ++
50. Good. ++

What you know: Range of motion is limited in elbow flexion. ***Priorities:*** Gain range of motion in flexion and then work for strength.

51. Not appropriate at this time. – –
52. Athlete has achieved full flexion. ++
53. Not appropriate at this time. – –
54. Appropriate. ++
55. Not necessary. –
56. Appropriate. ++
57. Athlete has achieved full extension. ++
58. This is helpful. ++
59. Okay. ++
60. Not appropriate at this time. – –
61. This is helpful. ++
62. Appropriate. ++
63. This is helpful. ++
64. This is helpful. ++

What you know: Athlete's strength is improving. ***Priorities:*** Gain strength in all ranges of motion.

65. Good. The athlete's strength is at full strength. ++
66. Not appropriate at this time. –
67. Strength is at 95 per cent of the other elbow. ++
68. Appropriate. ++
69. Inappropriate. – –
70. Appropriate. ++
71. Appropriate. ++
72. Inappropriate. – –
73. Appropriate. ++
74. Not necessary for this athlete. – –
75. Strength is greatly improved. ++
76. Good. ++

What you know: Athlete has good strength. ***Priorities:*** Get athlete prepared for return to activity.

77. Athlete wants an explanation. – –
78. She does fine, with no pain and without reservation. ++
79. Okay. ++
80. Good. ++
81. Okay. ++
82. Okay. ++
83. Athlete is unhappy. – –
84. Okay. ++

What you know: Athlete has been returned to activity. ***Priorities:*** Continue to ice after activity.
Passing-point total: 73

Problem 14

1. Do you have a prescription? – –
2. He says that it makes his shoulder throb. –
3. He points to the tip of his shoulder. ++
4. Not necessary. – –
5. Not necessary. –
6. Not necessary. – –
7. Okay. ++
8. Not necessary. – –
9. Do you have a prescription? – –
10. Not helpful. –
11. Do you have a prescription? – –
12. Athlete feels comfortable. ++
13. Not necessary at this time. –
14. You are placed on suspension. – –
15. It has full range of motion already. – –
16. Not necessary. – –
17. Not necessary. – –

What you know: An athlete with a rotator cuff injury has pain and decreased strength. Ice and electrical stimulation help with the pain. ***Priorities:*** Increase strength.

18. Pain decreases. ++
19. Athlete has no difficulty. ++
20. Not necessary. – –
21. Athlete has no difficulty with the exercise. ++
22. Okay. ++
23. Okay. ++
24. Okay. ++
25. Okay. ++
26. Okay. ++
27. Okay. ++
28. Okay. ++
29. Okay. ++
30. Okay. ++

What you know: Athlete has fair strength. ***Priorities:*** Begin light throwing with progression of strength.

31. Okay. ++
32. Okay. ++
33. Not appropriate. – –
34. Okay. ++
35. Okay. ++
36. Strength improves. ++
37. Okay. ++
38. Okay. ++
39. Okay. ++
40. Strength improves. ++
41. Okay. ++
42. Strength improves to full strength. ++

What you know: Full strength of the rotator cuff. ***Priorities:*** Increase distance of throws.

43. Inappropriate at this time. –
44. Okay. +
45. Inappropriate at this time. –
46. Okay. ++
47. Okay. ++
48. Inappropriate at this time. –
49. Okay. ++
50. Okay. ++
51. Okay. ++
52. Okay. ++

What you know: Strength is full. ***Priorities:*** Continue to increase distance of throws.

53. Okay. ++
54. Okay. ++
55. Okay. ++
56. Okay. ++
57. Okay. ++
58. Okay. ++
59. Okay. ++
60. Not necessary. – –

What you know: Athlete has full strength and has no difficulty throwing at 90 feet. ***Priorities:*** Continue to increase distance of throws.

61. Appropriate. ++
62. Athlete says this causing shoulder to be sore. 0
63. Appropriate. ++
64. Okay. ++
65. Okay. ++
66. Not appropriate at this time. – –
67. Okay. ++
68. Okay. ++
69. Athlete has full range of motion and flexibility. ++

What you know: Athlete has no difficulty throwing at 125 feet. ***Priorities:*** Increase distance of throws.

70. Appropriate. ++
71. Okay. ++
72. Appropriate. ++
73. Okay. ++
74. Okay. ++
75. Okay. ++
76. Okay. ++
77. Okay. ++
78. Okay. ++

What you know: Athlete has no difficulty throwing at 150 feet. ***Priorities:*** Return athlete to practice. ***Passing-point total:*** 77

Problem 15

1. Not necessary. – –
2. Not necessary. – –
3. Not necessary. – –
4. Not necessary. – –
5. Not necessary. – –
6. Not necessary. – –
7. Not necessary. – –
8. Not necessary. – –
9. Not necessary. – –
10. Not necessary. – –
11. Good idea. ++
12. Good idea. ++
13. Not necessary. – –
14. Not necessary. – –

What you know: Need a wrestling conditioning program for the off-season; at this point no exercises is necessary. ***Priorities:*** Determine baseline of fitness.

15. Not necessary. – –
16. Not necessary. – –
17. Not necessary. – –
18. Not necessary. – –
19. He has decreased strength in the triceps. ++
20. He has decreased strength in his calves. ++
21. Wrestler has normal flexibility. ++
22. Not necessary. – –
23. He runs a mile in seven and one half minutes. ++
24. Not necessary. – –
25. It is slightly decreased from in-season. ++
26. Not necessary. – –
27. He has decreased power. ++
28. He has lifted for his chest, quadriceps, and hamstrings. ++

What you know: Athlete has decreased total power and has decreased strength in his calves. ***Priorities:*** Increase power and strength in calves, along with general strengthening.

29. Okay. +
30. Okay. +
31. Good idea. ++
32. Good idea. ++
33. Power improves. ++
34. Not necessary at this time. – –
35. Okay. +
36. Okay. +
37. Incorrect. – –
38. Okay. +
39. Good idea. ++
40. Okay. +
41. Okay. +
42. Power improves. ++
43. Power improves. ++
44. Power improves. ++
45. Okay. +
46. Okay. +
47. Okay. +
48. Okay. +
49. Okay. +
50. Okay. ++
51. Okay. +
52. Okay. +
53. Okay. +
54. Okay. +
55. Okay. +
56. Okay. +
57. Okay. +
58. Okay. +
59. Okay. +
60. Okay. +
61. Power improves. ++

What you know: Power improves and calves strength is improved. ***Priorities:*** Work on a pre-season fitness program.

62. Not necessary at this time. – –
63. Okay to get started. +
64. Okay, since he is maintaining. +
65. Not necessary at this time. – –
66. Okay. +
67. Okay. +
68. Not necessary at this time. – –

What you know: Athlete is getting in aerobic and anaerobic shape. ***Priorities:*** Work on an in-season program.

69. Not necessary at this time. –
70. Not necessary at this time. –
71. Good. ++
72. Athlete does well with this. ++
73. Good. ++
74. Good. ++
75. Good. ++
76. Not necessary at this time. –
77. Good. ++
78. Okay. +
79. Good idea. ++

What you know: Athlete has reached peak physical condition. ***Priorities:*** Maintain athlete's fitness level. ***Passing-point total:*** *55*

Problem 16

1. He says no. 0
2. He says no. ++
3. He says he chose not to. +
4. Inappropriate. – –
5. He says he really doesn't know. +
6. He is not uncomfortable. 0
7. He says just let it rest and some icing. ++
8. He says no. +
9. Inappropriate. – –
10. Inappropriate. – –
11. Two weeks earlier. ++
12. Inappropriate. – –

What you know: Athlete has a two week old low back strain. ***Priorities:*** Assess the extent of injury.

13. His range is 0 to 80 degrees. +
14. Inappropriate. – –
15. Range of motion is normal. ++
16. His range is 0 to 20 degrees. +
17. Not necessary. – –
18. Not necessary. – –
19. His range is 0 to 45 degrees. +
20. His range is 0 to 45 degrees. +
21. Not necessary. – –
22. Not necessary. – –
23. Not necessary. – –
24. His range is 0 to 35 degrees. ++
25. His range is 0 to 35 degrees. ++
26. Range of motion is normal. ++
27. His range is 0 to 30 degrees. +

What you know: Range of motion is normal. ***Priorities:*** Continue to assess the extent of injury.

28. Not necessary. – –
29. Not necessary. – –
30. Not necessary. – –
31. Not necessary. – –
32. Not necessary. – –
33. Not necessary. – –
34. Not necessary. – –
35. Not necessary. – –
36. It is normal. ++
37. Not necessary. – –
38. Not necessary. – –
39. Not necessary. – –
40. Not necessary. – –

What you know: Quadriceps lumborm flexibility is normal. ***Priorities:*** Stretch the body in preparation for perform golf skills.

41. Appropriate. ++
42. Not necessary. – –
42. Appropriate. ++
43. Appropriate. ++
44. Appropriate. ++
45. Appropriate. ++
46. Not necessary. –
47. Appropriate. ++
48. Appropriate. ++

What you know: Stretching is normal. ***Priorities:*** Swinging clubs and prevention of reoccurrence.

49. Appropriate. ++
50. Not necessary. – –
51. Appropriate. ++
52. Not necessary. – –
53. Appropriate. ++
54. Appropriate. ++
55. Appropriate. ++
56. Not necessary. –

What you know: Athlete has no pain with golf swings. ***Priorities:*** Give preventive stretching and exercises.

57. These are helpful. ++
58. Not necessary. – –
59. Appropriate. ++
60. Not necessary. – –
61. Appropriate. ++
62. Not necessary. – –
63. Appropriate. ++
64. Not necessary. – –
65. Inappropriate. – –
66. Not necessary. – –
67. Not necessary. – –

What you know: Athlete is ready to play golf. ***Priorities:*** Monitor as necessary. ***Passing-point total:*** 39

Problem 17

1. He says, "This is hockey" but doesn't remember getting hit. +
2. He says he can't remember anything, but a couple of other guys also feel the same way. ++
3. There is no pain. 0
4. "I don't remember getting hit." – –
5. He says he feels dizzy and has a headache. ++
6. He says he can still play. –
7. It's open. – –
8. Athlete is unhappy with this question since the dizziness just occurred. –
9. There is no pain. –
10. No treatment has been given. – –
11. Rarely. +
12. "Many times, but not like this." –
13. He says no. +
14. He says he ate like a horse: pasta, chicken salad, pizza, French fries, nachos and cheese, pop, cookies, steak, baked potato, chips, and a banana. +
15. No swelling seen. – –
16. There is none. +
17. "It happened gradually over the first period." ++
18. Unnecessary. – –
19. You are in the locker room. – –
20. Unnecessary. – –
21. Several players indicate they feel the same way. ++
22. Athlete says no. +
23. He is conscious. – –
24. No one has, but several members indicate they feel dizzy and nauseous, too. ++

What you know: An athlete and several other players feel dizzy and nauseous. ***Priorities:*** Determine the cause of the illness or injury.

25. Not necessary. – –
26. Not necessary. – –
27. The only food they have in common is French fries but only two people ate at the same place. +
28. Unnecessary. – –
29. Unnecessary. – –
30. Athletes complain of some difficulty, but all are breathing normally. ++
31. Unnecessary. – –
32. Unnecessary. – –
33. They are on the way. ++
34. Unnecessary. – –
35. Unnecessary. – –
36. Unnecessary. – –
37. Unnecessary. – –

What you know: The athletes have some breathing difficulty, and the emergency medical system has been activated. ***Priorities:*** Treat the athletes.

38. Unnecessary. – –
39. Unnecessary. – –
40. Unnecessary. – –
41. It is cool but players feel better. ++
42. Unnecessary. – –
43. It is normal. 0
44. Athletes do not feel better. –
45. Unnecessary. – –

What you know: Athletes feel better outside of ice arena. ***Priorities:*** Get athletes to hospital and determine the source of the problem and warn others.

46. Not necessary. – –
47. It tastes good but doesn't make the athlete feel better. – –
48. Athlete does not feel better. – –
49. He says no and you need to forfeit if you don't continue the game. +
50. Good idea. ++
51. The athlete feels worse. – –
52. You begin to feel dizzy. – –
53. Athlete does not feel better. – –
54. Athlete does not feel better. – –
55. He goes, but unwillingly. 0
56. They go, but unwillingly. 0

What you know: Athletes go to the hospital. ***Priorities:*** Determine the cause.

57. Incorrect. – –
58. Incorrect. – –
59. Correct. ++
60. Incorrect. – –
61. Incorrect. – –
62. Incorrect. – –
63. Incorrect. – –
64. Incorrect. – –

What you know: The arena has carbon monoxide poison leak. ***Priorities:*** Arena should determine the source of the leak and evacuate the arena. ***Passing-point total:*** 20

Problem 18

1. You arrive but don't find the athlete. +
2. Nobody knows. 0
3. Improper. – –
4. Not necessary. –
5. The athlete is located at the mid-point of the race. ++
6. Inappropriate at this time. – –
7. She is from the Pioneers. +
8. It has a flat tire and cannot be driven. –
9. The color is purple. +
10. That is helpful. ++

What you know: A Pioneer athlete is injured in the middle of the race. ***Priorities:*** Get to the athlete and determine severity of injury.

11. Unnecessary. –
12. Unnecessary at this time. –
13. Nobody knows. 0
14. Improper. – –
15. Not appropriate. – –
16. You do not find the athlete. – –
17. Not appropriate. – –
18. Athlete is not found. 0
19. Improper. – –
20. She says no. +
21. Nobody knows what you are talking about. 0
22. She says, "Just one girl. But don't worry: her parents have her." +
23. Coach says she is just lazy and has never finished a race. +

24. Unnecessary. – –
25. The coach points to a section of the course. +
26. Not appropriate. – –

What you know: The injured athlete has left the area where she was injured and is with her parents. ***Priorities:*** Get to the athlete and determine the need to give assistance.

27. She is alert but refuses to talk with you. 0
28. The ambulance arrives. +
29. You find her in a van off the course. +
30. You can't get to athlete. – –
31. The parent responds, "You did not come when we asked for you. You'll not touch my daughter." +
32. You cannot get to the athlete. – –
33. Parent refuses to respond. +
34. They refuse. +
35. She starts screaming at you. –
36. They say she was having difficulty breathing. +
37. Inappropriate. – –

What you know: You have found the athlete who may have difficulty breathing, but her parents refuse your care. ***Priorities:*** Get the paramedics involved to try and get permission to treat.

38. Nobody responds. 0
39. Inappropriate. – –
40. Appropriate. ++
41. The person does not understand why they are here. +
42. They refuse. 0
43. They cite confidentiality. +
44. She is at the finish line. +
45. The person gives it to you but seems unsure of the reasoning. +
46. You find the Pioneer coach. +
47. Not appropriate. – –

What you know: Emergency medical technicians have taken over but you cannot get any information regarding the condition of the athlete. ***Priorities:*** Gather as much information as possible for documentation.

48. She says it is Cindy Jones. +
49. She says, "No. She has problems at every race, so I just ignore her." +
50. Okay. +
51. She is not available. 0
52. The coach does not know. 0
53. You gain a little weight, but don't solve the problem. –
54. The coach does not know. 0
55. It does not make your afternoon easier. –
56. Great. ++
57. Not effective. 0
58. It is an incorrect phone number. 0
59. Nobody tells you. 0

What you know: You have documented what you can. ***Priorities:*** Return to race coverage and inform those needing to know about a possible litigation

60. The athletic director wants to know what is wrong with the athlete. +
61. Good. +
62. The athletic director calls the Pioneer Middle school, and is given no information. 0
63. No real value. 0
64. Insignificant to resolution. 0
65. They cite client confidentiality. –
66. He refuses. –

What you know: It is not possible to determine the athletes illness or injury. ***Priorities:*** Prevention of such situations again.

67. She says that looks nice. +
68. Good idea. ++
69. Good. +
70. Good. +
71. You have six people including yourself. ++
72. The athletic director refuses. –
73. Good idea. ++
74. It is hard to predict this far in advance. –
75. Okay. +
76. Okay. +
77. Okay. 0
78. Not necessary. – –

79. Good choice. ++
80. There are several chained areas for which you do not have keys. +
81. Not helpful. –
82. Good idea. ++
83. There is no money. –
84. Not necessary. – –
85. Okay. +
86. It's near the finish. ++
87. It's the same as the last race. ++
88. Not appropriate at this time. –
89. It's near the finish. +
90. Not necessary. – –
91. Not necessary. – –
92. Not necessary at this time. –
93. Excellent. ++

What you know: You have a new plan that has been tested. ***Priorities:*** Cover the meet.
Passing-point total: 37

Problem 19

1. Inappropriate. – –
2. He has a headache. ++
3. Inappropriate. – –
4. Inappropriate. – –
5. Inappropriate. – –
6. He indicates he was hit in the lip by the ball. ++
7. Inappropriate. – –
8. Inappropriate. – –
9. Inappropriate; athlete dies; go to the next question. – –
10. Athlete is conscious. ++
11. He says his lip hurts. ++
12. He's on all fours and has blood dripping from his mouth. ++

What you know: A baseball player got hit in the mouth and is conscious and bleeding. ***Priorities:*** Check for an airway obstruction.

13. All teeth are in place. ++
14. Inappropriate. – –
15. Inappropriate. – –
16. Inappropriate. – –
17. Inappropriate. – –
18. Inappropriate. – –

What you know: There's no airway obstruction. ***Priorities:*** Stop the bleeding and determine the extent of the injury.

19. Inappropriate. – –
20. Inappropriate at this time. 0
21. Inappropriate. – –
22. This slows the bleeding down. ++
23. Inappropriate. – –
24. All bones are fine. ++
25. Inappropriate, please go to the next question. – –
26. Laceration of the lip likely from teeth going into the lip. +
27. Inappropriate, at this time. 0
28. Inappropriate. – –

What you know: Bleeding is slowing. ***Priorities:*** Determine the extent of the injury.

29. Inappropriate. – –
30. Equal and reactive. ++
31. Inappropriate, at this time. 0
32. Inappropriate. – –
33. Inappropriate. – –
34. Inappropriate. – –
35. Inappropriate. – –
36. He does not know, and he does not remember getting hurt. ++
37. He has none. ++
38. He's not. ++
39. He can balance without difficulty with his eyes open or closed. ++
40. Have athlete take a few warm-up tosses and swing a bat. – –

What you know: Athlete has a head injury. ***Priorities:*** Monitor the athlete.

41. Inappropriate – –
42. Appropriate. ++
43. Appropriate. ++
44. Inappropriate. – –
45. Appropriate. ++
46. Inappropriate. – –
47. Inappropriate. – –
48. Inappropriate. – –
49. Inappropriate. – –
50. Okay. 0

51. Inappropriate. – –
52. Inappropriate. – –
53. Appropriate. ++
54. Parent insists on taking him. ++

What you know: Athlete has a head injury and is going home with his parents. ***Priorities:*** Call the parents in the morning to determine the physician's diagnosis. ***Passing-point total:*** 27

Problem 20

1. Not necessary, but if you want to, that's fine. 0
2. He says he has had it for a couple weeks and now there are more. ++
3. Not necessary. – –
4. Excellent choice. ++
5. He says he borrowed his little brother's comb. +
6. Not necessary at this time. – –
7. Not necessary. – –
8. Okay. +
9. Not necessary at this time. –
10. Not necessary. – –
11. He has several well-defined red circular patches. He also has some small bald patches with scaling along his hairline. ++

What you know: The athlete has slow progressing skin condition in his hairline that may have been shared via a comb. ***Priorities:*** Determine the type of condition and if it spreads.

12. Okay. +
13. Good choice. +
14. That would be helpful. ++
15. Not necessary. 0
16. Not necessary. 0

What you know: It's a fungal infection. ***Priorities:*** Get athlete to physician for assessment and medication.

17. Inappropriate. – –
18. Not necessary. – –
19. This is helpful. ++
20. Going a little overboard. 0
21. Not necessary. – –
22. Might be helpful. +
23. Not necessary. – –
24. Not necessary. – –
25. Not necessary. – –
26. The other schools appreciate the contact. +
27. The nurse appreciates the information. ++
28. This is helpful for the team. ++
29. This is very helpful. ++
30. Not necessary. – –
31. Not necessary. – –
32. Not necessary. – –
33. Not necessary. – –
34. You don't find any. ++
35. Not necessary. – –

What you know: The athlete has a fungus and determining if others have it is important. ***Priorities:*** Education of athlete to ensure he does not transfer skin disorder.

36. Inappropriate. – –
37. Inappropriate. – –
38. Inappropriate. – –
39. He says he will. +
40. He agrees he made a mistake. ++
41. You better slow down. – –
42. The physician indicates athlete can return. ++

What you know: The athlete can return and you have educated him. ***Priorities:*** Start an educational program before next years' season to prevent transmission of skin or communicable diseases. ***Passing-point total:*** 21

Bibliography

The following textbooks and resources have been recommended for use as a study guide for the certification examination. You do not need to get all of them, but make sure you have several that are general in nature and a couple in each domain that are specific.

Many of the following references have been recommended by the National Athletic Trainer's Association Board of Certification. If you intend to use these references to study from, begin early. Some of these references have been used within this program as a cross-reference.

1. American Academy of Ophthalmology. 1982. The *Athlete's Ophthalmology and Sports.* San Francisco: American Academy of Ophthalomology.
2. American Academy of Orthopedic Surgeons. 1991. *Athletic Training and Sports Medicine.* 2nd ed. Park Ridge, IL: American Academy of Orthopaedic Surgeons.
3. American College of Sports Medicine. 1992 ACSM *Health Fitness Facility Standards and Guidelines.* Champaign, IL: Human Kinetics.
4. American College of Sports Medicine. 1997. *ACSM Exercise Management for Persons with Chronic Diseases* and Disabilities. Champaign, IL: Human Kinetics.
5. American College of Sports Medicine. 2000. ACSM *Guidelines for Exercise Testing and Prescription.* 6th ed. Philadelphia: Lippincott Williams and Wilkins.
6. American Red Cross. 1993. *Community First Aid & Safety.* St. Louis: Mosby-Year Book, Inc.
7. American Red Cross. 1993. *CPR for the Professional Rescuer.* Stay Well.
8. Anderson, Marsha and Susan Hall. 1995. *Sports Injury Management.* Baltimore: Williams and Wilkins.
9. Anderson, Marsha and Susan Hall. 1997. *Fundamentals of Sports Injury* Management. Philadelphia: Lippincott Williams and Wilkins.
10. Andrews, J., G. Harrelson and K. Wilk. 1991. *Physical Rehabilitation of the Injured Athlete.* 2nd ed. Philadelphia: WB Saunders.
11. Arnheim, Daniel. 1989. *Modern Principles of Athletic Training.* 7th ed. St. Louis: Times Mirror/Mosby.
12. Arnheim, Daniel. 1991. *Essentials of Athletic* St. Louis: Times Mirror/Mosby.
13. Arnheim, Daniel and William Prentice. 2000. *Principles of Athletic Training.* 10th ed. Boston: McGraw-Hill.
14. Baeche, T. and R.W. Earle. 2000. *Essentials of Strength Training and Conditioning.* 2nd ed. NSCA. Champaign, IL: Human Kinetics.

15. Baley, James A., and D. L. Matthews. 1984. *Law and Liability in Athletics, Physical Education and Recreation*. Boston: Allyn and Bacon, Inc.
16. Bates. Barbara, M.D. 1983. A *Guide to Physical Examination*. 3rd ed. Philadelphia: JB Lippincott Company.
17. Cartwright, Lorin. 1995. *Preparing for the Athletic Trainers' Certification Examination*. Champaign, IL: Human Kinetics.
18. Cartwright, Lorin and W. Pitney. 1999. *Athletic Training* for *Student Assistants*. Champaign, IL: Human Kinetics.
19. Clarkson, Hazel. 2000. *Musculoskeletal Assessment: Joint Range of Motion and Manual Muscle Strength*. 2nd ed. Philadelphia: Lippincott Williams and Wilkins.
20. Ethicon. 1999. *Wound Closure Manual*. Sommerville: Ethicon, Inc.
21. Gallaspy, James and Doug May. 1996. *Signs and Symptoms of Athletic Injuries*. St. Louis: CV Mosby.
22. Gallup, Elizabeth. 1995. Law *and the Team Physician*. Champaign, IL: Human Kinetics.
23. Grant, H.D., R.H. Murray, J.D. Bergeron. 1994. *Emergency* Care. 6th ed. Englewood Cliffs: Prentice Hall.
24. Greenfield, Bruce. 1993. *Rehabilitation of the Knee: A Problem-Solving Approach*. Philadelphia: F.A. Davis Co.
25. Griffin, James E. and T.C. Karselis. 1982. *Physical Agents for Physical Therapists*. 2nd ed. Springfield: Thomas Books.
26. Hall, Susan. 1995. *Basic Biomechanics*. 3rd ed. Boston: McGraw-Hill.
27. Hegarty, Vincent. 1988. *Decisions in Nutrition*. St. Louis: Times Mirror/Mosby.
28. Heil, John. 1993. *Psychology of Sport injury*. Champaign, IL: Human Kinetics.
29. Hoppenfeld, Stanley. 1976. *Physical Examination of the Spine and Extremities*. New York: Appleton-Century Crofts.
30. Howley, Edward T. and B. Don Franks. 1992. *Health Fitness Instructor's Handbook*. 2nd ed. Champaign, IL: Human Kinetics.
31. Jenkins, D.B. 1998. *Hollinghead's Functional Anatomy of the Limbs and Back*. 7th ed. Philadelphia: W.B. Saunders.
32. Kendall, F.P., McCreary, E.K. and P.G. Provance. 1993. *Muscles: Testing and Function*. 4th ed. Baltimore: Williams and Wilkins.
33. Kettenback, Ginge. 1990. *Writing SOAP* Notes. Philadelphia: F.A. Davis Co.
34. Kibler, W. Ben. 1990. *The Sports Preparticipation Fitness Examination*. Champaign, IL: Human Kinetics Publishers.
35. Kissner, Carolyn and Lynn Allen Colby. 1985. *Therapeutic Exercise: Foundations and Techniques*. Philadelphia: F.A. Davis Co.
36. Knight, Kenneth L. 1990. *Clinical Experiences in Athletic Training*. Champaign, IL: Human Kinetics.
37. Knight, Kenneth. 1995. *Cryotherapy in Sport Injury Management*. Champaign, IL: Human Kinetics.
38. Konin, J.G., D.L. Wikesteing, and J.A. Isear. 1997. *Special Test for Orthopedic Examination*. Thorofare, NJ: SLACK, Inc.
39. Konin, J.G. 1997. *Clinical Athletic Training*. Thorofare: Slack, Inc.
40. Magee, D.J. 1987. *Orthopedic Physical Assessment*. 2nd ed. Philadelphia: WB Saunders.

41. *MBM 2000 Buyers* Guide. 2000. Micro Bio-Medics. Inc.
42. McArdle, Willam, F. Katch and V. Katch. 2000. *Essentials of Exercise Physiology*. Baltimore: Lippincott Williams and Wilkins.
43. McArdle, William, F. Katch and V. Katch. 1981. *Exercise Physiology: Energy, Nutrition, and Human Performance*. Philadelphia: Lea and Febiger.
44. McAtee, R.E. 1993. *Facilitated Stretching*. Champaign, IL: Human Kinetics.
45. Michlovitz, S. 1996. *Thermal Agents in Rehabilitation*. 3rd ed. Philadelphia: F.A. Davis Co.
46. Moore, K., and A.F. Dalley. 1999. *Clinically Oriented Anatomy* . 4th ed. Baltimore: Lippincott Williams and Wilkins.
47. Mottram, D.R. 1988. *Drugs in Sport*. Champaign, IL: Human Kinetics Publishers.
48. NATA. 1997. CEU *Requirements and Appeal Process Brochure*. Dallas: NATA.
49. NATA. 1997. *Study Guide for Management of Bloodborne Pathogens by Athletic Trainers*. Champaign, IL: Human Kinetics.
50. NATA. 1998 "Code *of Ethics*." Dallas: National Athletic Trainers' Association, Inc.
51. NATA. 1998. NATA *Membership Standards, Eligibility Requirements, and Membership Sanctions and Procedures*. Dallas: NATA, Inc.
52. NATA. 1999. Sexual *Harassment What Every Athletic Trainer Should* Know. Dallas: NATA.
53. NATA. Fall 2000. *NATA Recommendations for Lightning Safety*. Dallas: NATA, Inc.
54. NATA. December 2000. NATA News. Dallas: NATA, Inc.
55. National Athletic Trainers' Association Board of Certification, Inc. Spring 1993. *Certification Update*. Dallas: NATA.
56. NATABOC. January 1997. *Recertification Requirements and Policies Professional Practice and Disciplinary Procedures*.
57. NATABOC. August 1997. *Credentialing Information Entry-Level Eligibility Requirements*.
58. NATABOC. 1999. *Role Delineation Study: Athletic Training Profession*. 4th ed. Raleigh: Columbia Assessment Services, Inc.
59. NATABOC. January 2000. *Continuing Education Guidelines, 2000-2002*. Omaha: NATABOC.
60. NATABOC. *Certification Update*. Summer 2000. Omaha: NATABOC.
61. NATABOC. March 16, 2000. *NATABOC Frequently Asked Questions*. Omaha: NATABOC.
62. NATABOC. June 23, 2000. *Disciplinary Process*. Omaha: NATABOC.
63. NATABOC. June 23, 2000. *Requirements to Maintain Certification*. Omaha: NATABOC.
64. NATABOC. June 23, 2000. *Standards of Professional Practice*. Omaha: NATABOC.
65. O'Donaghue, Donald. 1976. *Treatment of Injuries to Athletes*. 3rd ed. Philadelphia: WB Saunders.
66. Perrin, David. 1995. *Athletic Taping and Bracing*. Champaign, IL: Human Kinetics.
67. Perrin, David. 1993. *Isokinetic Exercise and Assessment*. Champaign, IL: Human Kinetics.

68. Peterson, M., and K. Peterson. 1988. *Eat to Compete: A Guide to Sports Nutrition*. Chicago: Year Book Medical.
69. Prentice, William. 1994. *Therapeutic Modalities in Sports Medicine*. 3rd ed. St. Louis: CV Mosby.
70. Prentice, William. 1999. *Therapeutic Modalities in Sports Medicine*. 4th ed. Boston: McGraw-Hill.
71. Prentice, William. 1990. *Rehabilitation Techniques in Sports Medicine*. St. Louis: CV Mosby.
72. Prentice, William. 1999. *Rehabilitation Techniques in Sports Medicine*. 3rd ed. Boston: McGraw-Hill.
73. Rankin, James and C. Ingersoll. 1995. *Athletic Training Management: Concepts and Applications*. Boston: McGraw-Hill.
74. Ray, Richard. 1994. *Management Strategies in Athletic Training*. Champaign, IL: Human Kinetics.
75. Ray, Richard and D.M. Wiese-Bjornstal. 1999. *Counseling in Sports Medicine*. Champaign, IL: Human Kinetics.
76. Ray, Richard. 2000. *Management Strategies in Athletic Training* 2nd ed. Champaign, IL: Human Kinetics.
77. Rothstein, J.M,. S.H. Roay, and S.L. Wolf. 1998. *The Rehabilitation Specialist's Handbook*. Philadelphia: F.A. Davis Co.
78. Roy, S. and R. Irvin. 1983. *Sports Medicine: Prevention, Evaluation, Management and Rehabilitation*. Englewood Cliffs: Prentice Hall.
79. Salter, Robert B. 1970. *Textbook of Disorders and Injuries of the Musculoskeletal System*. Baltimore: Williams and Wilkins.
80. Starkey, Chad and J. Ryan. 1996. *Evaluation of Orthopaedic and Athletic Injuries*. Philadelphia: F.A. Davis Co.
81. Starkey, Chad. 1999. *Therapeutic Modalities*. 2nd ed. Philadelphia: F.A. Davis Co.
82. Thomas, C.L. ed. 1997. *Taber's Cyclopedic Medical Dictionary*. 18th ed. Philadelphia: Philadelphia: F.A. Davis Co.
83. Thomas, J., and J.K. Nelson. 1996. *Research Methods in Physical Activity*. 3rd ed. Champaign, IL: Human Kinetics.
84. Tippett, S.R., and M.L. Voight. 1995. *Functional Progression for Sports Rehabilitation*. Champaign, IL: Human Kinetics.
85. Torg, Joseph, J. Vegso, and E. Torg. 1987. *Rehabilitation of Athletic Injuries: An Atlas of Therapeutic Exercise*. Chicago: Year Book Medical Publishers, Inc.
86. Torg, Joseph. 1991. *Athletic Injuries to the Head, Neck and* Face. 2nd ed. St. Louis: CV Mosby.
87. Williams, Melvin. 1988. *Nutrition for Fitness and Sport*. Dubuque: Wm. C. Brown.
88. Wilmore, J.H. and D.L. Costill. 1999. *Physiology of Sport and Exercise*. 2nd ed. Champaign, IL: Human Kinetics.
89. Zachazewski, J.E., D.J. Magee, and W.S. Quillen. 1996. *Athletic Injuries and Rehabilitation*. Philadelphia: W.B. Saunders.
90. Zarins, B., Andrews, J.R., and W.G. Carson. 1985. *Injuries to the Throwing Arm*. Philadelphia: WB Saunder Co.
91. Ziegler, T. 1997. *Management of Bloodborne Infection in Sport: A Practical Guide for Sports Healthcare Providers and Coaches*. Champaign, IL: Human Kinetics.

About the Author

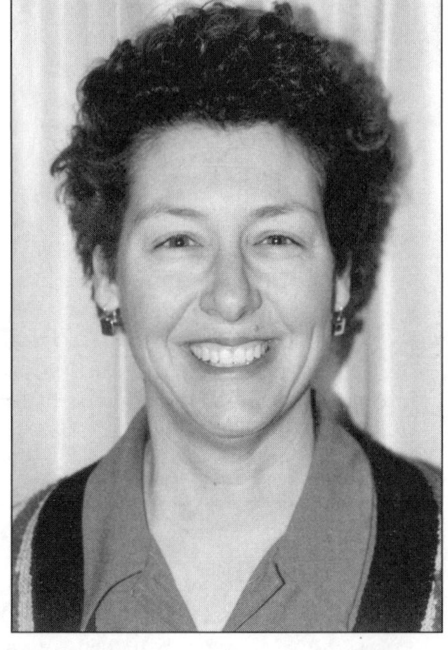

Lorin Cartwright, MS, EMT, ATC, CAA, is the athletic director at Pioneer High School in Ann Arbor, Michigan. Since she became certified as an athletic trainer in 1980, Lorin has put her knowledge and experience to good use by helping numerous students study for and pass the National Athletic Trainers' Association (NATA) certification exam. Not only has she served as an examiner for several NATA exams, which has given her insights into common errors students make on the test, but she also has taken numerous certification tests herself and learned firsthand about test-taking strategies and skills.

Lorin received an MS in education from the University of Michigan in 1981. She is a member of NATA, the National Interscholastic Athletic Administration Association, and the Michigan Athletic Trainers' Society. She earned the NATA Distinguished Service Award in 1999 and in 2000 and became a certified athletic administrator (CAA).

In addition to being a frequent speaker at NATA national clinical symposiums, Lorin is the author of several articles on injury prevention. In 1994 she became the first woman, as well as the first high school athletic trainer, to be elected president of District IV of NATA. She is also the coauthor of *Athletic Training for Student Assistants*. In 2001, she was honored as part of the inaugural class of distinguished alumni in residence at Grand Valley State University.